Nonintubated Thoracic Surgery

Editors

VINCENZO AMBROGI
TOMMASO CLAUDIO MINEO

THORACIC SURGERY CLINICS

www.thoracic.theclinics.com

Consulting Editor
M. BLAIR MARSHALL

February 2020 • Volume 30 • Number 1

ELSEVIER

1600 John F. Kennedy Boulevard • Suite 1800 • Philadelphia, Pennsylvania, 19103-2899

http://www.thoracic.theclinics.com

THORACIC SURGERY CLINICS Volume 30, Number 1
February 2020 ISSN 1547-4127, ISBN-13: 978-0-323-68129-2

Editor: John Vassallo (j.vassallo@elsevier.com)
Developmental Editor: Laura Fisher

Thoracic Surgery Clinics (ISSN 1547-4127) is published quarterly by Elsevier Inc., 360 Park Avenue South, New York, NY 10010-1710. Months of publication are February, May, August, and November. Business and editorial offices: 1600 John F. Kennedy Boulevard, Suite 1800, Philadelphia, PA 19103-2899. Periodicals postage paid at New York, NY, and additional mailing offices. Subscription prices are $393.00 per year (US individuals), $623.00 per year (US institutions), $100.00 per year (US students), $460.00 per year (Canadian individuals), $806.00 per year (Canadian institutions), $100.00 per year (Canadian students), $225.00 per year (international students), $480.00 per year (international individuals), and $806.00 per year (international institutions). Foreign air speed delivery is included in all Clinics' subscription prices. All prices are subject to change without notice. **POSTMASTER:** Send address changes to Thoracic Surgery Clinics, Elsevier Health Sciences Division, Subscription Customer Service, 3251 Riverport Lane, Maryland Heights, MO 63043. **Customer Service (orders, claims, online, change of address): Telephone: 1-800-654-2452 (U.S. and Canada); 314-447-8871 (outside U.S. and Canada). Fax: 314-447-8029. E-mail: journalscustomerservice-usa@elsevier.com (for print support); journalsonlinesupport-usa@elsevier.com (for online support).**

Reprints. For copies of 100 or more, of articles in this publication, please contact Commercial Rights Department, Elsevier Inc., 360 Park Avenue South, New York, NY 10010-1710. Tel: 212-633-3874; Fax: 212-633-3820; E-mail: reprints@elsevier.com.

Thoracic Surgery Clinics is covered in *MEDLINE/PubMed (Index Medicus), EMBASE/Excerpta Medica, Science Citation Index Expanded (SciSearch®), Journal Citation Reports/Science Edition,* and *Current Contents®/Clinical Medicine.*

Contributors

CONSULTING EDITOR

M. BLAIR MARSHALL, MD, FACS
Associate Chief for Quality and Safety, Division of Thoracic Surgery, Brigham and Women's Hospital, Associate Professor of Surgery, Harvard Medical School, Boston, Massachusetts, USA

EDITORS

VINCENZO AMBROGI, MD, PhD
Department of Surgical Sciences, Tor Vergata University, Division of Thoracic Surgery, Tor Vergata University Policlinic, Rome, Italy

TOMMASO CLAUDIO MINEO, MD[†]
Department of Surgical Sciences, Tor Vergata University, Rome, Italy

AUTHORS

ANDREY AKOPOV, MD, PhD
Professor, Saint Petersburg, Russia

VINCENZO AMBROGI, MD, PhD
Department of Surgical Sciences, Tor Vergata University, Division of Thoracic Surgery, Tor Vergata University Policlinic, Rome, Italy

SERGIO BOLUFER, MD, PhD
Thoracic Surgery Department, Hospital General Universitario Alicante, Alicante, Spain

REBECCA CARR, MBBS
General Surgery Resident, Department of Surgery, Sinai Hospital of Baltimore, Baltimore, Maryland, USA

JIN-SHING CHEN, MD, PhD
Professor, Division of Thoracic Surgery, Department of Surgery, National Taiwan University Hospital, National Taiwan University College of Medicine, Taipei, Taiwan

PEI-HSING CHEN, MD
Division of Thoracic Surgery, Department of Surgery, National Taiwan University Hospital Yun-Lin Branch, Douliu City, Yun-Lin County, Taiwan

YA-JUNG CHENG, MD, PhD
Professor, Department of Anesthesiology, National Taiwan University Hospital, National Taiwan University College of Medicine, Taipei, Taiwan

JONG HO CHO, MD, PhD
Department of Thoracic and Cardiovascular Surgery, Samsung Medical Center, Sungkyunkwan University School of Medicine, Seoul, Korea

SOLANGE COX, MD
General Surgery Resident, Department of Surgery, Sinai Hospital of Baltimore, Baltimore, Maryland, USA

MARIA GALIANA-IVARS, MD
Anesthesiology Department and Surgical Critical Care Unit, Hospital General Universitario de Alicante, Alicante, Spain

[†]Deceased.

CARLOS GÁLVEZ, MD, PhD
Thoracic Surgery Department, Hospital General
Universitario de Alicante, Alicante, Spain

ELISA GÁLVEZ, MD, PhD
Medical Oncology, Hospital General
Universitario Elda, Elda, Alicante, Spain

DIEGO GONZALEZ-RIVAS, MD
Department of Thoracic Surgery, Coruña
University Hospital, Coruña, Spain

JIANXING HE, MD, PhD
Department of Thoracic Surgery, The First
Affiliated Hospital of Guangzhou Medical
University, State Key Laboratory of Respiratory
Disease, National Clinical Research Center for
Respiratory Disease, Guangzhou Institute of
Respiratory Health, Guangzhou, China

WAN-TING HUNG, MD
Attending Surgeon, Division of Thoracic
Surgery, Department of Surgery, National
Taiwan University Hospital, Taipei, Taiwan

MARK KATLIC, MD
Chairman, Department of Surgery, Sinai
Hospital of Baltimore, Baltimore, Maryland, USA

TAE HO KIM, MD
Department of Thoracic and Cardiovascular
Surgery, Samsung Medical Center,
Sungkyunkwan University School of Medicine,
Seoul, Korea

GABOR KISS, MD
Department of Anesthesia for Cardiothoracics
and Vascular Surgery, University Hospital Felix
Guyon, Allée des Topazes, Saint Denis,
Réunion, France

MIKHAIL KOVALEV, MD, PhD
Saint Petersburg, Russia

MARTA ORTEGA LAMAIGNÈRE
Surgical Nurse, Hospital General Universitario
de Alicante, Alicante, Spain

SHUBEN LI, MD, PhD
Department of Thoracic Surgery, The First
Affiliated Hospital of Guangzhou Medical
University, State Key Laboratory of Respiratory
Disease, National Clinical Research Center for
Respiratory Disease, Guangzhou Institute of
Respiratory Health, Guangzhou,
China

HENGRUI LIANG, MD
Department of Thoracic Surgery, The First
Affiliated Hospital of Guangzhou Medical
University, State Key Laboratory of
Respiratory Disease, National Clinical
Research Center for Respiratory Disease,
Guangzhou Institute of Respiratory Health,
Guangzhou, China

JUN LIU, MD, PhD
Department of Thoracic Surgery, The First
Affiliated Hospital of Guangzhou Medical
University, State Key Laboratory of
Respiratory Disease, National Clinical
Research Center for Respiratory Disease,
Guangzhou Institute of Respiratory Health,
Guangzhou, China

ELENA DÍEZ MAZO
Surgical Nurse, Hospital General Universitario
de Alicante, Alicante, Spain

MARCELLO MIGLIORE, MD, PhD, FETCS
Section of Thoracic Surgery, Department of
Surgery and Medical Specialities, University of
Catania, Policlinic University Hospital, Catania,
Italy

TOMMASO CLAUDIO MINEO, MD†
Department of Surgical Sciences, Tor Vergata
University, Rome, Italy

SERGIO BOLUFER NADAL, MD, PhD
Thoracic Surgery Department, Hospital
General Universitario de Alicante, Alicante,
Spain

JOSE NAVARRO-MARTÍNEZ, MD, EDAIC
Anesthesiology Department and Surgical
Critical Care Unit, Hospital General
Universitario de Alicante, Alicante,
Spain

THAMER ROBERT QAQISH, MD
Chief Resident, Department of Surgery, Sinai
Hospital of Baltimore, Baltimore, Maryland,
USA

MARÍA JESÚS RIVERA-COGOLLOS, MD
Anesthesiology Department and Surgical
Critical Care Unit, Hospital General
Universitario de Alicante, Alicante,
Spain

JULIO SESMA, MD
Thoracic Surgery Department, Hospital
General Universitario Alicante, Alicante, Spain

FEDERICO TACCONI, MD
Department of Surgical Sciences, Division of
Thoracic Surgery, Tor Vergata University
Hospital, Tor Vergata University, Rome,
Italy

RICCARDO TAJÈ, MS
Division of Thoracic Surgery, Tor Vergata
University Policlinic, Rome, Italy

XI WU, MD
Department of Anesthesia, The First
Affiliated Hospital of Guangzhou
Medical University, Guangzhou,
China

YANRAN ZHOU, MD
Department of Anesthesia, The First Affiliated
Hospital of Guangzhou Medical University,
Guangzhou, China

Contents

Nonintubated thoracic surgery (NITS) has a good safety record in experienced hands, but has pitfalls for beginners. The main aim of NITS is to keep the patient under spontaneous respiration, avoiding adverse effects, such as hypoxemia, hypercapnia, panic attacks, and finally conversion to general anesthesia. In this article, the safety aspects of anesthesia for NITS is discussed based on data from the literature and personnel clinical experiences.

Nonintubated video-assisted thoracoscopic surgery for the treatment of primary and secondary pneumothorax was first reported in 1997 by Nezu. However, studies on this technique are few. Research in the past 20 years has focused on the perioperative outcomes, including the surgical duration, length of hospital stay, and postoperative morbidity and respiratory complication rates, which appear to be better than those of surgery under intubated general anesthesia. This study provides information pertaining to the physiologic, surgical, and anesthetic aspects and describes the potential benefits of nonintubated thoracoscopic surgery for the management of primary and secondary spontaneous pneumothorax.

Video-assisted thoracic surgery has considerably improved the care of the thoracic surgical patient. Patients are able to leave the hospital sooner and experience less pain with equal oncologic outcomes when compared with open surgery. Nonintubated thoracic surgery has more recently been applied in the management of both benign and malignant pleural effusions. This article provides the general thoracic surgeon a detailed description on how to manage pleural effusions using video-assisted thoracoscopic surgery in a nonintubated patient. Surgical techniques and pearls are also presented.

Chest infection is a health care problem in many regions of the world, and pleural empyema is the most common type of surgical chest infection. In the past decennium, the introduction of nonintubated surgery and uniportal video-assisted thoracic surgery changed considerably surgical treatment of pleural empyema. Although the advantages seem evident, the need for randomized controlled trials is necessary to confirm the usefulness. Moreover, in the future, an education and training program for thoracic surgeons and anesthesiologists would allow increasing the number of awake surgical options in caring for patients with stages II to III empyema.

Interstitial lung diseases are a heterogeneous group with diffuse parenchymal lung disease. Because most patients with interstitial lung diseases have impaired pulmonary function, the risks of thoracic surgery are an important issue when considering surgical lung biopsy. The nonintubated video-assisted thoracoscopic surgery lung biopsy for interstitial lung disease is a safe and feasible option in carefully selected patients with interstitial lung disease.

Wedge resection in peripheral lung cancer is considered a suboptimal procedure. However, in elderly and/or frail patients it is a reliable and safer alternative. This procedure can be easily performed under nonintubated anesthesia, allowing the recruitment of patients considered otherwise marginal for a surgical treatment. Nonintubated anesthesia can reduce lung trauma, operative time, postoperative morbidity, hospital stay, and global expenses. Furthermore, nonintubated anesthesia produces less immunologic impairment and this may affect postoperative oncological long-term results. Wedge lung resection through nonintubated anesthesia can be performed for diagnosis with higher effectiveness given the similar invasiveness of computed tomography–guided biopsy.

 Video content accompanies this article at http://www.thoracic.theclinics.com.

Thoracic surgery has evolved into minimally invasive surgery, in terms of not only surgical approach but also less aggressive anesthesia protocols and lung-sparing resections. Nonintubated anatomic segmentectomies are challenging procedures but can be safely performed if some essentials are considered. Strict selection criteria, previous experience in minor procedures, multidisciplinary cooperation, and the 4 cornerstones (deep sedation, regional analgesia, oxygenation support and vagal blockade) should be followed. Better outcomes in postoperative recovery, including resumption of oral intake, chest tube duration, and hospital stay, and low complication and conversion rates, are encouraging but should be checked in larger multicenter prospective randomized trials.

Nonintubated video-assisted thoracoscopic surgery (VATS) lobectomy to treat lung cancer has gained attention in recent decades, but there is very little literature on this topic. This review aims to explore the state-of-the-art, recent progress, and future prospects of this method. Its feasibility and safety have been demonstrated, and its potential benefits are faster postoperative recovery and fewer intubation-related complications. Nonintubated VATS lobectomy is a feasible and safe alternative for lung cancer treatment. This work provides information for those who would like to start using this technique and want a more comprehensive understanding of nonintubated VATS lobectomy.

Nonintubated anesthesia is feasible and might be associated with shorter surgery time and shorter hospitalization for tracheal/carinal resection and reconstruction. Only case reports and a few small retrospective series study were conducted to evaluate nonintubated anesthesia for tracheal/carinal resection and reconstruction; no randomized control trials exist. Further exploration should focus on selection of optimal candidates and prospective validation.

The article describes an anesthetic management strategy for resection of the cervical trachea due to benign stenosis without using an endotracheal tube. The strategy includes: (1) insertion of an airway stent in the stenotic area, (2) insertion of a supraglottic airway device (SGAD), and (3) advancing a jet ventilation catheter through the SGAD. The stent is removed during surgery together with the resected part of the trachea. The technique of nonintubated tracheal resection allows the surgeon to work most comfortably and helps the anesthesiologist properly maintain the patient's vital functions in the operating room.

Nonintubated video-assisted thoracoscopic surgery programs have gradually spread all over the world. The benefits are based on less invasiveness and earlier recovery. However, complications may appear. For the correct prevention and management of all these potentially critical situations, the principles of crisis resource management (CRM) must be followed. They should also include clinical simulation as a tool to generate different scenarios to improve teamwork. The purpose of this special issue is to appraise and summarize the design, implementation, and efficacy of simulation-based CRM training programs for a specific surgery, including the management of specific surgical and medical critical scenarios.

Nonintubated thoracic surgery arose as supplemental evolution of minimally invasive surgery and is gaining popularity. A proper nonintubated thoracic surgery unit is mandatory and should involve surgeons, anesthesiologists, intensive care physicians, physiotherapists, psychologists, and scrub and ward nurses. Surgical training should involve experienced and young surgeons. It deserves a step-by-step approach and consolidated experience on video-assisted thoracic surgery. Due to difficulty in reproducing lung and diaphragm movements, training with simulation systems may be of scant value; instead, preceptorships and invited proctorships are useful. Preoperatively, patients must be fully informed. Effective intraoperative communication with patients and among the surgical team is pivotal.

THORACIC SURGERY CLINICS

SERIES OF RELATED INTEREST

Surgical Clinics
http://www.surgical.theclinics.com

Surgical Oncology Clinics
http://www.surgonc.theclinics.com

Advances in Surgery
http://www.advancessurgery.com

Preface

In my life, all my efforts were, are and will be inspired by the passion for surgery and the devotion to university institutions.
— *Tommaso Claudio Mineo (1945-2018)*

In March 2001, at the old Sant'Eugenio Hospital in Rome, Professor Mineo and I performed our first awake thoracic operation for a peripheral pulmonary nodule on an 82-year-old man. He was a heavy smoker with severe chronic obstructive pulmonary disease and diabetes. The operation was preceded by thorough preparation to dispel skepticism among colleagues and to obtain official permission from our internal review board. Nothing would have been possible without the frequent consultation with the group of anesthesiologists directed by Professor Alessandro Fabrizio Sabato (1944-2016), pioneer of therapy of the pain in Italy, and assisted by his pupil, Mario Dauri, presently director of the Anesthesiology Department at Tor Vergata Policlinic University. They helped us consider the feasibility of the procedure and the management of all potential side effects. Thanks to God, the operation was straightforward; the recovery was rapid, and all parties were satisfied: patient, surgeons, referring physicians, and administration as well. We were so satisfied with the procedure that we captured the event with a photograph (**Fig. 1**).

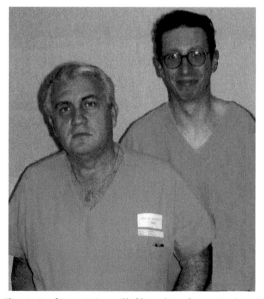

Fig. 1. Professor Mineo (*left*) and Professor Ambrogi (*right*) after their first nonintubated operation in 2001.

Professor Mineo had known Dr Eric Carlens, the creator of the double lumen tube, during his time in Stockholm in the 1970s. He learned directly from him the use of this tube and acknowledged the noteworthy advantages of this technique. The introduction of one-lung ventilation through selective intubation was welcomed as a brilliant solution to safely perform thoracic surgery with a deflated lung. Indeed, for decades, transthoracic procedures have been exclusively conducted under this anesthesiologic approach. However, the numerous drawbacks of this technique pushed surgeons to research new and less-invasive alternatives.

The advent of video-assisted procedures and the most recent successful development of the uniportal approach have significantly reduced hospital stay, morbidity, mortality, and postoperative pain with better cosmesis while conserving the same efficacy of the widest open accesses. This surgical revolution and the introduction of new anesthesiologic drugs and operative tools led to further minimization of the anesthesiologic impact of the procedure with the development of nonintubated surgery.

The first objective of this anesthesiologic/surgical modality is the reduction of all postoperative complications due to classic intubated general anesthesia operations, promoting a quicker and more durable recovery. As the second objective, this technique allows the recruitment of a subset of patients with comorbidity otherwise excluded from surgery. The third objective is the reduction of operative expenses and hospital-stay costs inducing a progressive interest among health system institutions.

Nonintubated awake thoracic surgery is becoming more reputable and attractive. At present, a significant number of surgical procedures are performed at an increasing rate in institutions throughout the world. So far, after 20 years of experience, is it possible to affirm that thoracic operations under nonintubated anesthesia are as complete and safe as those under general anesthesia and one-lung ventilation? To better answer this question, I involved many colleagues and friends, each one having a high level of expertise in this field, in this project. All of them are renowned scientists devoted to this particular approach. This issue of *Thoracic Surgery Clinics* would not have been possible without their cooperation and friendship. Thanks to these contributions, we will increase awareness of this amazing approach.

Thorac Surg Clin 30 (2020) xi–xii
https://doi.org/10.1016/j.thorsurg.2019.09.004
1547-4127/20/© 2019 Published by Elsevier Inc.

Finally, I would address this issue to surgical residents and young surgeons. I well know that they are most interested in this innovative field, and for this reason, a specific article in this issue is dedicated to them.

There is a final point that I feel is very important to mention. On December 2, 2018, Professor Tommaso Claudio Mineo, coeditor of this issue, passed away after a short illness. He was also a cultured and eclectic man, as well as a Roman Catholic Christian devoted to the Virgin Mary, to Whom he dedicated numerous books.

Until his last moments, even on his deathbed, Professor Mineo was speaking with his pupils about science, academy, and religion. He asked me to finish the issue that he conceived and would have carried out by himself had he been able to.

Now, I am very proud to say that, thanks to all the contributors' efforts, we completed the issue.

This is the best way to honor your memory, my dear Professor. Thank you so much again.

Vincenzo Ambrogi, MD, PhD
Department of Surgical Sciences
Tor Vergata University
Rome, Italy

Division of Thoracic Surgery
Tor Vergata University Policlinic
Policlinico Tor Vergata University
Viale Oxford 81
Rome 00133, Italy

E-mail address:
ambrogi@med.uniroma2.it

Technical Issues and Patient Safety in Nonintubated Thoracic Anesthesia

Gabor Kiss, MD

KEYWORDS

• Safety • Nonintubated thoracic surgery • Awake • Spontaneous respiration • Epidural anesthesia
• Regional anesthesia • Hypnosis • Conversion

KEY POINTS

- Knowing indications and contraindications to nonintubated thoracic anesthesia (NITS) is imperative for patient selection and safety.
- Key aim of NITS is to keep the patient under spontaneous respiration avoiding hypoxemia, hypercapnia, panic attacks, and finally conversion to general anesthesia.
- Attention must be payed to pitfalls in premedication, regional anesthesia techniques, spinal opioids, blockage of the cough reflex, and intraoperative sedation.
- A multimodal approach and opioid-free anesthesia for NITS does not replace an effective local anesthesia or a good working regional anesthesia block.
- Stepwise correction of reversible causes of hypoxemia is necessary before a thoroughly planned conversion.

INTRODUCTION

In experienced hands, nonintubated thoracic surgery (NITS) achieves an acceptable safety profile. However, NITS is full of pitfalls for beginners. The technique may be adopted either in patiens who are fully awake or under light sedation. In both cases, patients breathe spontaneously without any definitive airway intubation, although some kind of respiratory assistance (eg, manual ventilation or even laryngeal mask) may be set up on occasion. In essence, the main aim of NITS is to keep the patient under spontaneous respiration and avoid adverse effects, such as hypoxemia, hypercapnia, panic attacks, and finally conversion to general anesthesia.

In this article, the safety aspects of anesthesia for NITS are discussed based on data from the literature and on personal clinical experience.

SAFETY

Thoracic surgery under general anesthesia shows equivalent surgical results compared with awake thoracic surgery and is correlated with lower mortality and morbidity.[1–8]

Several studies conclude that NITS is superior to thoracic surgery under general anesthesia by reducing operating room time and the incidence of postoperative respiratory infections and acute respiratory distress syndrome, thus lowering mortality rate and improving perioperative outcomes with less

Disclosure: The author has nothing to disclose.
Department of Anesthesia for Cardiothoracics and Vascular Surgery, University Hospital Felix Guyon, Allée des Topazes, Saint Denis F-97400, Réunion, France
E-mail address: gaborkiss2001@hotmail.com

need for nursing, lower costs, and shorter hospital stays.[9]

ACQUIRING KNOWLEDGE

Only trained staff should participate during NITS. Education and training programs in thoracic surgery with nonintubated patients is needed before starting NITS, ideally in either high-volume centers or, even better, under proctorship.[10] To acquire experience in awake thoracic surgery, surgeons and anesthesiologists should begin with minor procedures in strictly selected patients and in a cooperative environment with all the necessary background knowledge of NITS.[11]

A good way to start is to perform NITS first in simple cases and then to proceed to more complex cases step by step. It should be kept in mind that strict coordination and vigilance are the keys for successful patient management for NITS.

CONTRAINDICATIONS

Knowing the contraindications to NITS is imperative for patient selection. Contraindications can be divided into surgical and anesthetic contraindications (**Box 1**).

From an anesthesiology point of view, the following conditions should be regarded as major contraindications to NITS: (1) contralateral phrenic nerve paralysis, (2) expected difficult airway, (3) persistent cough or excessive airway secretion, (4) high risk of aspiration, (5) severe cardiopulmonary dysfunction, and (6) patients with a body mass index (BMI) of >30 kg/m^2 (or >35 kg/m^2).[11–14] In fact, the higher the BMI, the more the anatomic disadvantage of a higher mediastinum-to-chest ratio.[14] Furthermore, an elevated diaphragm, which is very common in these patients, puts them at a higher risk of impaired intraoperative ventilation and atelectasis. Consequently, as morbidly obese patients carry more risks for intraoperative respiratory depression, nonintubated procedures should not be attempted in these patients.[14] Spine deformities and coagulopathy, although not major contraindications to NITS in themselves, do not allow safe insertion of thoracic epidural catheter, so that alternative analgesia techniques should be considered in these cases.

From a surgical point of view, NITS should be avoided in patients with expected extensive pleural adhesions and previous pulmonary resection. NITS in patients scheduled for major resection should be limited to those with stage I non-small-cell lung cancer. In addition, the following conditions may also dictate some

---

Box 1
Contraindications to NITS quoted in literature

General contraindications

- Refusal of the patient
- Inexperienced and poorly cooperative surgical team
- Critical ASA status
- BMI greater than 30 or 35 kg/m^2

Anesthetic contraindications

- Difficult airways
- ppoFEV1 less than 30%
- Chest deformity
- Pulmonary infection
- Severe cardiopulmonary dysfunction
- Hemodynamically unstable patient
- Coagulopathy
- Contralateral phrenic nervous paralysis
- Persistent cough or excessive airway secretion
- Gastric reflux

Surgical contraindications

- Coagulopathy
- Extensive pleural adhesion
- Prior pulmonary resection or previous ipsilateral chest surgery
- Clinical stage N2 lung cancer
- Foreseeable surgical difficulties
- Bleeding of pulmonary artery

Abbreviations: BMI, body mass index; ppoFEV1, predicted postoperative forced expiratory volume in first second.

---

caution (see **Box 1**): American Society of Anaesthesiologists status greater than 2, a tumor size of greater than 6 cm, and other foreseeable surgical difficulties complicating vascular dissection or incomplete fissure. However, Elkhouly and Pompeo[15] have reported that NITS might still be feasible in experienced hands, even with conditions that were regarded as major contraindications in early literature. These include pleural adhesions, previous thoracic surgery, neoadjuvant chemotherapy or radiation, central lesions, and chest wall or vascular involvement (**Box 2**). Furthermore, in contrast to contraindications quoted in the literature, some authors also noticed that the application of NITS can be extended to high-risk patients with poor performance status,[16] compromised respiratory function, and to those older than 80 years.[16,17]

Box 2
Relative contraindications to NITS who are considered to be safe in experienced hands and indicated for NITS

- Diffuse pleural adhesions
- Previous thoracic surgery
- Neoadjuvant chemotherapy or radiation
- Central lesions
- Chest wall or vascular involvement
- High-risk patients with poor preoperative performance status
- Compromised respiratory function
- Elderly patients greater than 80 years
- Terminally ill but stable patients

INDICATIONS

From a surgical point of view, there are subgroups of patients who are more likely to benefit from NITS. NITS is ideally suited for patients with pneumothorax in whom there is a risk of increasing air collection, making ventilation conditions more difficult in case of intubation with one-lung ventilation[2,16,18,19] Also, patients with a high risk for ventilator dependency, such as lung transplant candidates, patients with severe neuromuscular disease, patients who have undergone lung transplantation[20] and pregnant women,[21] are better candidates for NITS than for general anesthesia (**Box 3**). Unfortunately, these patients also have a higher probability of conversion, so that a contingency plan should be well discussed and prepared. In the literature, good results have been reported in these patients using NITS with various analgesia techniques.[17,22]

Box 3
Good indications for NITS

- Pleural effusion
- Empyema
- Pathologies with chronic collapse of the operated lung
- Pneumothorax
- Lung transplantation
- Pregnancy
- History of difficult intensive care unit weaning from ventilation
- Fast-track thoracic surgery

In other categories of patients, the advantages of NITS are less clear. However, there is a suggestion that it might reduce postoperative adverse events because of less inflammatory impact on the airways. In fact, compartmental airway inflammation has a pivotal role in the development of perioperative complications after general anesthesia, and it may occur even when protective ventilation strategies are adopted.[22–26] Patients with complex pleural effusion and empyema are already prone to lung collapse, because they tolerate surgical pneumothorax during spontaneous one-lung breathing very well. For this reason, these patients may also be good candidates for NITS.[13,27]

In addition, patients who have already undergone a long weaning process from a ventilator in their past medical history could also be considered for NITS. This is sometimes requested by the patients themselves, when they are willing to avoid such an unpleasant and traumatic experience.[17] In general, NITS might be applied as a part of an integrated fast-track with the objective of shortening hospitalization as much as possible.[28]

SELECTION

Patient selection for NITS is crucial to avoid tricky pitfalls. Contraindications and indications, as described in **Boxes 1–3**, constitute the first criteria for careful patient selection. Patient refusal is a total contraindication for NITS and any persuasion attempts should be avoided. Both the surgeon and anesthetist should have full agreement on offering NITS. Preoperatively, patients and their relatives must be fully informed on the pros and cons of NITS, including the risk of conversion to general anesthesia. This should be reported in the consent form to avoid any misunderstandings.

PREMEDICATION

Ideally, one should always use drugs that can be antagonized, such as benzodiazepines with flumazenil. Some patients do not want any premedication,[17] and this needs to be respected. Alternatively, preoperative sessions of hypnosis could also replace pharmaceutical premedication, thereby avoiding respiratory depression induced by premedication.[29]

MONITORING

The following standard monitoring should be applied in preparation of NITS (**Box 4**): routine monitoring with electrocardiogram, pulse oximetry, noninvasive blood pressure and noninvasive end tidal CO_2 ($ETCO_2$) connected to either a nasal oxygen cannula or an oxygen mask. At least 2 intravenous lines for the operation have to be inserted. One of them is for fluid replacement and the other one for drug administration, mainly for cardiovascular support if necessary. For more difficult cases, for example, patients with severe comorbidities, invasive radial artery monitoring may be needed to control oxygen saturation and to prevent excess hypercapnia. In addition, in high-risk patients, a central venous line is to be inserted, in preference into a femoral vein, to avoid respiratory distress and complications in the thorax region. In the case of thoracic epidural anesthesia, a urinary catheter should be inserted to avoid retention.

Although the algorithm of the bispectral index does not accurately predict an unconscious state,[30] it can be helpful as an adjunct.[12]

All equipment and drugs for conversion in the case of emergency should also be prepared in advance.

During surgery, except in cases of severe chronic obstructive pulmonary disease (COPD), in which high-flow oxygen could lead to respiratory depression, high-flow oxygen nasal prongs up to 40 L/min can be administered to stabilize the patient and achieve an oxygen saturation of more than 90%.[31] It is critical to maintain the threshold level of the mean arterial pressure above 65 mm Hg and oxygen saturation greater than 90%. When mean arterial pressure falls below 65 mm Hg and/or systolic arterial pressure below 90 mm Hg, fluids should be administered if needed, otherwise vasoactive drugs are to be given. In cases in which epidural-induced hypotension remains resistant to ephedrine, neosynephrine/phenylephrine should be infused. If more than 1,200 μm/min of neosynephrine is required, it can be replaced by

noradrenaline. If oxygen saturation is below 90%, noninvasive ventilation should be applied to recruit the lungs in the spontaneously breathing patient.[17]

EPIDURAL AND INTRATHECAL OPIOID ANALGESIA

To achieve the optimal spread of anesthesia, which is in relation to the planned level of surgical incision, the anatomic puncture level of the epidural block should be discussed with the surgeon in advance. Puncture level is usually between T3 and T7. It is important to note that the volume of anesthesia solution that is administered also depends on the length of the incision (the longer the incision the more volume injected) and also varies with the size and weight of the patient.[17]

For obtaining a quick onset of an anesthetic block, lidocaine and chirocaine are the first choices. For long-lasting analgesic effect, administer ropivicaine (7.5 mg/mL) or bupivacaine (5 mg/mL), or higher concentrations. One has to avoid local anesthetic solutions of low concentration, because the patient might feel intrathoracic manipulations, which could lead to pain or panic attacks.[17] Moreover, local anesthetic of high concentration could lead to a motor block, which could contribute to decreasing the tidal volume. However, in my personal experience, high concentrations of ropivacaine 0.75% did not impair spontaneous respiration, even in patients with severe respiratory disease undergoing NITS.[17]

Providing a continuous epidural perfusion is safer than top-up bolusses through the epidural catheter to keep the patients constantly pain-free throughout the procedure and also provide better hemodynamic stability.

The main side effects of thoracic epidural anesthesia are urinary retention and hypotension (**Box 5**). In addition, liberal administration of intravenous fluids in the case of epidural-induced hypotension could lead to wet lung. Therefore, vasopressors are preferable to obtain a mean arterial pressure of at least 65 mm Hg. Hemodynamic instability caused by hypotension is a common side effect of thoracic epidural anesthesia, although it is rarely observed with continuous paravertebral block (**Box 6**).[32] The paravertebral block offers the advantages of a unilateral block without bilateral sympathectomy and lower incidence of hypotension. There is also less urinary retention and fewer neurologic complication. In contrast to epidural anesthesia, the paravertebral block also provides an alternative in cases of sepsis, coagulation disorders, neurologic disorders and difficult vertebral anatomy when an epidural is difficult to perform. In this regard, Baidya and colleagues[33] conclude that thoracic paravertebral block may be as effective as thoracic epidural analgesia for postthoracotomy pain relief and is also associated with fewer complications. The paravertebral block

offers the advantages of a unilateral block without bilateral sympathectomy and urinary retention. There are also fewer neurologic complications. In contrast to epidural anesthesia, the paravertebral block also provides an alternative in cases of sepsis, coagulation disorders, neurologic disorders, and difficult vertebral anatomy when an epidural is difficult to perform. However, as reported by Beyaz and colleagues[34], it must be mentioned that equally to thoracic epidural anesthesia, paravertebral block can also lead to a total spinal block. In each case, the benefits of epidural anesthesia have to be counterbalanced with its risks, such as epidural hematomas, spinal nerve injury, phrenic nerve palsy, and inadvertent high anesthetic level (see **Boxes 5** and **6**).[33] In particular, a risk of neurologic complication owing to epidural has been reported as 0.07%.[35] The safety profile of epidural anesthesia was also evaluated by Kang and colleagues,[36] who concluded that serious complications, such as epidural hematoma (0.02%) and postoperative neurologic deficits (1.12%), were very rare. Generally speaking, compared with thoracic surgery under general anesthesia, NITS under thoracic epidural anesthesia provides more advantages than disadvantages, especially in high-risk patients, such as diffuse interstitial lung fibrosis and limb girdle myopathy.[17]

Some attention should be paid to intrathecal opioid administration for thoracic surgery. This strategy has been shown to be effective for postoperative pain control after thoracotomy and also been effectively used in cardiac surgery.[37–40] However, there are pros and cons concerning adding opiates into continuous infusion of local anesthetics. The main advantage is the additive analgesic effect. On the other hand, there is a certain risk of respiratory depression.[41] Ouerghi and colleagues[42] have shown that magnesium sulfate intrathecally added to morphine and fentanyl reduces postoperative analgesia requirements in patients undergoing pulmonary resection, and prolongs spinal opioid analgesia without increasing opioid side effects. Gwirtz et al., in a study by of nearly 6000 patients who underwent many types of surgical specialties—including thoracic surgery—reported that the safety record of intrathecal opioid administration for acute postoperative pain was good, with a low incidence of side effects and complications. Pruritus was the most common (37%) side effect; other side effects were minor and easily managed. Respiratory depression was the least common side effect (3%), which was never life-threatening and always responsive to treatment with naloxone.[43]

A randomized prospective study showed that a combination of paravertebral block and intrathecal

---

Box 6
Comparison between thoracic epidural anesthesia and thoracic paravertebral block for NITS

Thoracic epidural anesthesia:

- Hemodynamic instability as a result of hypotension
- Bilateral block with possibility for bilateral sympathectomy
- Contraindicated in the case of sepsis or coagulation disorders
- Difficult to perform in the case of difficult vertebral anatomy
- Risk of epidural hematomas
- Risk of spinal nerve injury
- Risk of phrenic nerve palsy
- Risk of inadvertent high anesthetic level
- Well-known technique with large clinical experience in the literature

Thoracic paravertebral block:

- Less hypotension than thoracic epidural anesthesia
- One sided surgery without bilateral block
- Unilateral block without bilateral sympathectomy
- Lower incidence of hypotension
- Lower incidence of urinary retention
- Feasible in the case of sepsis or coagulation disorders
- Feasible in the case of neurologic disorders
- Feasible in the case of difficult vertebral anatomy

opioid administration can be considered a satisfactory clinical alternative to thoracic epidural anesthesia for postthoracotomy pain relief.[44] In another similar study by Madi-Jebara and colleagues,[45] intrathecal opioid administration was not inferior compared with thoracic epidural infusions of fentanyl and bupivacain in terms of pain control and hemodynamic stability after thoracotomy. Nevertheless, to the best of my knowledge, there is at present no paper describing the use of intrathecal opioid administration for NITS in spontaneously breathing patients. Therefore, intrathecal opioid administration should not be applied alone and—at least—it should be combined with a paravertebral block as described in Dango and colleagues.[44]

REGIONAL ANESTHESIA

Regional anesthesia has the advantage to provide better hemodynamic stability compared with general anesthesia.[46] Muscular plane blocks (serratus anterior plane block, pectoral blocks type I and II, and erector spinae block) and intercostal nerve block are increasingly being used in thoracic surgery (**Box 7**). Regarding local infiltration of lidocaine and, because of its short action, one has to take into account that lidocaine is especially suitable for short-lasting surgery.[47–50]

Erector Spinae Block

The erector spinae block also has been used for pain relief in thoracotomy[51,52] and can be performed without ultrasound guidance. This block is presumed to be safe because of the absence of major neurovascular bundles and, akin to epidural block, it can be performed at nearly all levels of the spine.[52,53] However, the good erector spinae block safety records have been put into question by a case describing Harlequin syndrome associated with erector spinae block

---

Box 7
Regional anesthesia for NITS

- Thoracic epidural anesthesia
- Thoracic paravertebral block
- Serratus anterior plane block
- Pectoral nerve block (PECS) type I and II
- Erector spinae block
- Intercostal nerve block
- Intrapleural injection of lidocaine
- Interpleural blocks

---

owing to ipsilateral interruption of the autonomic pathway.[54]

Blocks of the Pectoral Nerves

Anesthesia of pectoral nerves type I blocks the lateral and medial pectoral nerves. Roy[55] has shown that pectoral block is effective as a motor block but not as a skin sensory block. Although pectoral nerve type I block combined with pectoral nerve II and serratus plane block has been successfully applied to awake spontaneously breathing patients undergoing videothoracoscopy,[56] because of a lack of controlled studies on pectoral nerve type I block, it should not be used as a sole regional anesthesia technique for awake patients.

Even though intercostal nerve blocks are frequently used for analgesia in thoracic surgery, one has to be aware of the rare possibility of a risk of total spinal block.[57]

In conclusion, before choosing a regional anesthesia technique, risk and benefit have to be balanced for each case. The general rule is doing simple anesthesia for simple surgery.[11] In general, anesthetic techniques should not go beyond the need for the surgical procedure.

In summary, studies have proven that thoracic epidural anesthesia, paravertebral and intercostal blocks, adapted to the type of surgery, are reliable to obtain complete intraoperative analgesia, even for awake patients without sedation. To avoid pain sensations and panic attacks, serratus anterior plane block and pectoral nerve type I blocks should not be relied on as sole anesthetic techniques for providing complete analgesia for awake thoracic surgery. Erector spinae block provides postoperative pain relief for thoracotomy, but there are no publications on its use for awake thoracic surgery.

OPIOID-FREE ANESTHESIA

Nonopiate anesthesia targeting multimodal pathways for pain, such as α-1 agonists (ie, clonidine or dexmedetomidine), N-methyl D-aspartate antagonists (eg, ketamine and magnesium), intravenous local anesthetic infusions (eg, lignocaine) combined with multimodal analgesia, including paracetamol and tramadol, have shown to be a useful adjunct to provide perioperative and postoperative analgesia, especially if regional anesthesia is suboptimal.[58] However, clonidine, which is also used as a treatment for hypertension, should not be combined with thoracic epidural anesthesia because of the risk of increasing epidural-induced hypotension.

In the case of a local or regional anesthesia technique, it should be kept in mind that a multimodal approach to intraoperative analgesia for awake spontaneously breathing patients, such as opioid-free anesthesia, does not replace an effective local anesthesia infiltration or a good working regional anesthesia block. In contrast to regional anesthesia, opioid-free anesthesia is not a means to provide full pain-free surgery while the patient remains awake.

COUGH REFLEX

Coughing cannot be blocked by epidural anesthesia or intercostal block. However, the cough reflex can be controlled by inhalation of aerosolized lidocaine[59] or application of a spray of lidocaine on the lung surface,[60] phrenic nerve block, stellate ganglion block, intravenous administration of opioids, and intrathoracic vagal block.[61]

Vagal nerve injury induced by infiltration for radio frequency ablation has led to abdominal complications, such as bloating, abdominal distention, or abdominal pain and satiety.[62] At present, to my knowledge, there are no reports in the literature on vagal nerve injury in NITS.

Stellate ganglion block is generally safe to perform, but there are some reports of severe complications, such as retropharyngeal hematomas leading to airway obstruction, 1 case report of quadriplegia secondary to pyogenic cervical epidural abscess and discitis and local anesthetics-induced toxicity.[63]

NONINVASIVE VENTILATION

In contrast to the vast majority of the patients who tolerate high-flow oxygen (15 L/min), patients with severe COPD do not tolerate high-flow oxygen. Assist ventilation can successfully reverse hypercapnia.[17] As reported, transient perioperative permissive hypercapnia (<55 mm Hg) does not require conversion to general anesthesia.[1,5,14] When high-flow oxygen administration does not correct a fall in oxygen saturation, one should not hesitate to apply positive end-expiratory pressure as high as necessary and as tolerated by the patient to counteract pressure exerted by intraabdominal contents on the diaphragm, thereby reversing lung atelectasis. Noninvasive positive pressure ventilation combined with epidural anesthesia for patients with compromised respiratory function has been applied with good results.[59,64]

INTRAOPERATIVE SEDATION

Intraoperative sedation might be necessary when patients become anxious and panic, or if surgical and anesthestic conditions are difficult. Advantages of sedation is blunting the cough reflex and movement from artificial pneumothorax.[65,66] However, sedation during NITS is associated with potential risks (Box 8), such as the occurrence of apnea. Therefore, short-acting and reversible anesthesia agents should be used for sedation, such as remifentanil, with an ultra-short half-life of 3 minutes. Propofol or ketamine are further options for sedation. Ketamine (starting with 0.1–0.5 mg/kg intravenously [IV] up to 1–2 mg/kg IV followed by 1–2 mg/kg/h ketamine) can also be used in patients with severe COPD because it maintains the functional residual capacity.[67]

Galvez and colleagues[31] obtained deep sedation in spontaneously breathing patients with remifentanil infusion of 0.05 to 0.1 µg/kg/min and intravenous bolus of 1 to 2 mg of midazolam. In a paper by Kiss and colleagues[17] patients remaining conscious during surgery had light sedation with propofol with a target plasma concentration between 0.5 and 2 µg/mL (Shneider)[17] and remifentanyl with a plasma concentration between 0.5 and 3 ng/mL (Minto).[17] One patient with severe COPD (forced expiratory volume in the first second 27%) and a history of difficult weaning from a ventilator, had been sedated with target-controlled infusion of propofol and had plasma concentrations at around 0.3 µg/mL and remifentanil of 0.3 to 0.7 ng/mL, which probably might have contributed or accentuated hypercapnia. Therefore, the above-proposed plasma levels of propofol and remifentanil should be interpreted as guide reference values rather than absolute clinical targets.

In the United States and in Europe, dexmedetomitine is licensed for surgical procedures where the patient remains fully conscious, a strategy that is termed awake sedation (European Medicine Agency, https://www.ema.europa.eu/en/medicines/human/EPAR/dexdor).

Box 8
The risk of sedation

- Silent aspiration with respiratory infection and pneumonia
- Decreased deglutition
- Decreased muscle tone of the auxiliary inspiratory muscles and the diaphragm
- Depression of spontaneous respiration
- Ketamine saliva production
- Hypercapnia of greater than 55 mm Hg with need for conversion to general anesthesia

Dexmedetomitine preserves respiratory functions but it can also decrease blood pressure and heart rate, a fact which has to be taken into account during selection of patients for this type of sedation. Nevertheless, a study by Lodenius and colleagues[68] concludes that dexmedetomitine-induced sedation reduces ventilatory responses to hypoxia and hypercapnia to a similar extent as sedation with propofol. Therefore, dexmedetomitine has to be applied with the same cautions as propofol because under sedation the swallowing reflex might be less functional and there is a risk of silent aspiration. Therefore, it is preferable to use anesthetics, such as ketamine, which preserves deglutition and have been shown to have a high safety profile.[67] Because the risks of gastroesophageal reflux are still present in a spontaneously breathing patient, the insertion of a laryngeal mask airway (the LMA Protector) allows the passage of a lubricated gastric tube to the stomach thereby allowing evacuation of gastric contents helping to prevent aspiration. The LMA Protector can even be inserted in the lateral position.[69]

Hypnosis

Hypnosis may also be an interesting tool, especially as far as swallowing reflex in patients undergoing nonintubated surgery is concerned. In fact, other than general benefits as relaxation and anxiety control, it does not alter swallowing at all. In the vast majority of patients, a preparatory protocol is needed to achieve better results by applying hypnosis[70] (following on from a personal conversation with Dr. John Butler from the Hypnotherapy Training International, London, UK). However, fast hypnotic induction can be achieved in some 30% of patients who are highly susceptible for hypnosis[71] and do not need specific preparation. Other than the effect on swallowing, hypnosis can also help avoid nausea and vomiting. Therefore, it may be applied as a tool to protect patients from aspiration pneumonia, a severe complication that may easily occur even in intubated patients, especially if a double lumen tube is used.[72–74]

CONVERSION TO GENERAL ANESTHESIA

In many NITS cases, adverse events are limited to just patient anxiety and panic, without any substantial change in cardiorespiratory parameters. If this is the case, the following steps should be made to reduce anxiety: reinsurance, explanation, and guaranteeing a calm environment in the operating room. If the patient is willing to do so, one can allow him to watch the operation on the video.

If these measures do not temper anxiety, stepwise sedation should be used. However, in the case of insufficient analgesia and inadequate sedation or other technical difficulties, conversion may be indicated (**Box 9**).

In some situations, before proceeding to conversion, especially to the end of surgery, intubation can be still avoided by correction of reversible causes of hypoxemia with the following steps[17]:

- Correction of hypoxia by titrating oxygen if tolerated up to a high oxygen flow to achieve an oxygen saturation of at least 90%
- Application of noninvasive ventilation in case if high oxygen flow is not sufficient to obtain an oxygen saturation of at least 90%
- Sedation and application of a Guedel tube. If tolerated, noninvasive ventilation can also be established
- Sedation with a laryngeal mask airway combined with assisted spontaneous ventilation
- Definitive conversion to general anesthesia in case of persistent hypoxemia

---

Box 9
Indications for conversion to general anesthesia

Surgical difficulties:

- Unsatisfactory lung collapse
- Major bleeding
- Dense adhesion
- Significant mediastinal movement
- Complications during surgery
- Lack of progression of surgery over a significant lapse of time

Anesthetic difficulties:

- Insufficient analgesia
- Inadequate sedation
- Respiratory acidosis (respiratory rate above 30 bpm)
- Hypercapnia leading to coma
- Refractory hypoxemia
- Excessive mediastinal and diaphragmatic movement
- Deep respiratory movements
- Unstable hemodynamics
- Ineffective vagal block with persistent cough
- Panic attack
- Voluntary desire of the patient

In some cases, rebreathing mechanism of expired air into the dependent lung can produce some degree of hypoxemia and hypercapnia.[75]

In 2014, Hung and coworkers defined criteria for conversion from NITS to general anesthesia. These include: development of uncontrollable respiratory acidosis with respiratory rate above 30 bpm, refractory hypoxemia (oxygen saturation under 90% or mean arterial oxygen pressure under 60 mm Hg), deep respiratory movements, unstable hemodynamic status, ineffective vagal block with persistent cough, panic attack, voluntary desire of the patient, or severe bleeding requiring thoracotomy.[1,7,13,76] As mentioned before, transient perioperative permissive hypercapnia (<55 mm Hg) usually does not require conversion to general anesthesia.[1,5,14] Nevertheless, Lan Lan and colleagues[77] state that permissive hypercapnia is not infinitely permissive, and one should not to just rely on $EtCO_2$, because this can underestimate the real $Paco_2$ concentration. Therefore, blood gas analysis is required in these situations. In addition, excessive hypercapnia, excessive mediastinal, diaphragmatic movement, and potential complications during technical steps of the surgery also indicate conversion to general anesthesia.[11,61,78]

Typical surgical conditions whereby a timely conversion is required are the presence of calcified perivascular lymph nodes or extensive scarring, as well as diffuse dense pleural adhesions or major bleeding limiting a clear visualization and exposure of the pulmonary vessels.[79] Decaluwe and colleagues[80] have shown that up to 84% of conversions for operative complications during videothoracoscopy are because of inadvertent vascular bleeding. However, the rate of conversion in case of bleeding depends on the technical skills and experience of the surgeon.

Conversion to general anesthesia should not be regarded as a failure but as another step of patient management. The rate of conversion varies from 0% up to 13% in the literature.[8,50,81,82] Experienced teams described a conversion rate of 1.6% to orotracheal intubation.[11] In general, priority is given to anesthesia first and then to surgery. The surgeon can quickly close the open wound with 1 thick silk stitch and a large surgical drape. An additional bedsheet, which is put on the operating table before the patient is transferred on to it, allows to pull and to tilt the patient from the lateral to the dorsal position.[83] Intubation in the lateral decubitus position is technically challenging and potentially leads to critical complications.[78] A semilateral position or modified supine position would be safer. During conversion, the easiest, quickest, and safest option should be chosen for oral intubation and a single-lumen tube is usually the first choice. Once the airway is secured, a bronchial blocker can be used.[84] Nasal intubation that has been done successfully during conversion carries the risks of bleeding and should be avoided.[85]

Airways and Difficult Intubation

The airways is a major concern in NITS. In difficult intubations, a preoperative naso-fiberoptic examination shows whether awake NITS could be contraindicated. In case of conversion to general anesthesia, airway management could be increased stepwise by first starting with the insertion of a supraglottic airway device, which is also the first rescue tool to be applied according to protocols for difficult intubation.[86–88] A suspected difficult intubation is a relative contraindication to NITS and plays into the discussion of the risks benefice balance whether to avoid lung injury owing to mechanical ventilation. Moreover, difficult airway guidelines always propose to wake up the patient in case of failed intubation attempts and to keep him under spontaneous respiration.[87] The literature even recommends avoiding intubation in the case of a large mediastinal mass compressing upper airways as a result of inducing severe airway collapse not reversible with high positive end-expiratory pressure ventilation.[89–91] In addition, there are also reports that patients with signs of a difficult intubation have also been indicated for NITS under spontaneous breathing to avoid airway damage during intubation attempts and to respect the choice of the patient's preference for NITS under spontaneous breathing.[17]

ACKNOWLEDGMENTS

The author wants to express his sincere gratitude for the opportunity to contribute to the memory of Professor Tommaso Claudio Mineo, who died unexpectedly shortly after he initiated this project for a series of publications and personally invited him to participate. Despite his absence, he still remains one of the greatest specialists worldwide in nonintubated thoracic surgery. May his memory with his valuable and impressive work from his lifetime continued to be carried on for generations to come.

REFERENCES

1. Mineo TC, Pompeo E, Mineo D, et al. Awake nonresectional lung volume reduction surgery. Ann Surg 2006;243:131–6.

2. Noda M, Okada Y, Maeda S, et al. Is there a benefit of awake thoracoscopic surgery in patients with secondary spontaneous pneumothorax? J Thorac Cardiovasc Surg 2012;143:613–6.

3. Klijian AS, Gibbs M, Andonian NT. AVATS: Awake Video Assisted Thoracic Surgery–extended series report. J Cardiothorac Surg 2014;9:149.

4. Pompeo E, Tacconi F, Mineo TC. Comparative results of non-resectional lung volume reduction performed by awake or non-awake anesthesia. Eur J Cardiothorac Surg 2011;39:e51–8.

5. Pompeo E, Tacconi F, Frasca L, et al. Awake thoracoscopic bullaplasty. Eur J Cardiothorac Surg 2011;39:1012–7.

6. Tacconi F, Pompeo E, Sellitri F, et al. Surgical stress hormones response is reduced after awake videothoracoscopy. Interact Cardiovasc Thorac Surg 2010;10:666–71.

7. Pompeo E, Mineo D, Rogliani P, et al. Feasibility and results of awake thoracoscopic resection of solitary pulmonary nodules. Ann Thorac Surg 2004;78:1761–8.

8. Chen JS, Cheng YJ, Hung MH, et al. Nonintubated thoracoscopic lobectomy for lung cancer. Ann Surg 2011;254:1038–43.

9. Kiss G. Ethical, general and technical issue in anaesthesia for awake thoracic surgery in high risk patients. Surg Curr Res 2017;7(Suppl):5.

10. Park SY. Non-intubated thoracic surgery under thoracic epidural anesthesia. Korean J Anesthesiol 2017;70:235–6.

11. Wang ML, Galvez C, Chen JS, et al. Non-intubated single-incision video-assisted thoracic surgery: a two-center cohort of 188 patients. J Thorac Dis 2017;9:2587–98.

12. Ahn S, Moon Y, AlGhamdi ZM, et al. Korean J Thorac Cardiovasc Surg 2018;51:344–9.

13. Hung MH, Hsu HH, Cheng YJ, et al. Nonintubated thoracoscopic surgery: state of the art and future directions. J Thorac Dis 2014;6:2–9.

14. Tacconi F, Pompeo E, Fabbi E, et al. Awake video-assisted pleural decortication for empyema thoracis. Eur J Cardiothorac Surg 2010;37:594–601.

15. Elkhouly A, Pompeo E. Conversion to thoracotomy in thoracoscopic surgery: damnation, salvation or timely choice? Shanghai Chest 2018;2:2.

16. Mukaida T, Andou A, Date H, et al. Thoracoscopic operation for secondary pneumothorax under local and epidural anesthesia in high-risk patients. Ann Thorac Surg 1998;65:924–6.

17. Kiss G, Claret A, Desbordes J, et al. Thoracic epidural anaesthesia for awake thoracic surgery in severely dyspnoeic patients excluded from general anaesthesia. Interact Cardiovasc Thorac Surg 2014;19:816–23.

18. Noda M, Okada Y, Maeda S, et al. Successful thoracoscopic surgery for intractable pneumothorax after pneumonectomy under local and epidural anesthesia. J Thorac Cardiovasc Surg 2011;141:1545–7.

19. Shigematsu H, Andou A, Matsuo K, et al. Thoracoscopic surgery using local and epidural anesthesia for intractable pneumothorax after BMT. Bone Marrow Transplant 2011;46:472–3.

20. Sugimoto S, Date H, Sugimoto R, et al. Thoracoscopic operation with local and epidural anesthesia in the treatment of pneumothorax after lung transplantation. J Thorac Cardiovasc Surg 2005;130:1219–20.

21. Onodera K, Noda M, Okada Y, et al. Awake videothoracoscopic surgery for intractable pneumothorax in pregnancy by using a single portal plus puncture. Interact Cardiovasc Thorac Surg 2013;17:438–40.

22. Lohser J. Evidence-based management of one-lung ventilation. Anesthesiol Clin 2008;26:241–72.

23. Blank RS, Colquhoun DA, Durieux, et al. Management of one-lung ventilation: impact of tidal volume on complications after thoracic surgery. Anesthesiology 2016;124:1286–95.

24. Fernandez-Bustamante A, Frendl G, Sprung J, et al. Postoperative pulmonary complications, early mortality, and hospital stay following noncardiothoracic surgery: a multicenter study by the perioperative research network investigators. JAMA Surg 2017;152:157–66.

25. Canet J, Gallart L, Gomar C, et al, ARISCAT Group. Prediction of postoperative pulmonary complications in a population-based surgical cohort. Anesthesiology 2010;113:1338–50.

26. Agostini P, Cieslik H, Rathinam S, et al. Postoperative pulmonary complications following thoracic surgery: are there any modifiable risk factors? Thorax 2010;65:815–8.

27. Pompeo E. Awake thoracic surgery—is it worth the trouble? Semin Thorac Cardiovasc Surg 2012;24:106–14.

28. James JT. A new, evidence-based estimate of patient harms associated with hospital care. J Patient Saf 2013;9:122–8.

29. Potié A, Roelants F, Pospiech A, et al. Hypnosis in the perioperative management of breast cancer surgery: clinical benefits and potential implications. Anesthesiol Res Pract 2016;2016:2942416.

30. Medical Advisory Secretariat. Bispectral index monitor: an evidence-based analysis. Ont Health Technol Assess Ser 2004;4:1–70.

31. Galvez C, Navarro-Martinez J, Bolufer S, et al. Non-intubated uniportal left-lower lobe upper segmentectomy (S6). J Vis Surg 2017;3:48.

32. Pintaric TS, Potocnik I, Hadzic A, et al. Comparison of continuous thoracic epidural with paravertebral block on perioperative analgesia and hemodynamic stability in patients having open lung surgery. Reg Anesth Pain Med 2011;36:256–60.

33. Baidya DK, Khanna P, Maitra S. Analgesic efficacy and safety of thoracic paravertebral and epidural analgesia for thoracic surgery: a systematic review and meta-analysis. Interact Cardiovasc Thorac Surg 2014;18:626–35.

34. Beyaz SG, Özocak H, Ergönenç T, et al. Total spinal block after thoracic paravertebral block. Turk J Anaesthesiol Reanim 2014;42:43–5.

35. Giebler RM, Scherer RU, Peters J. Incidence of neurologic complications related to thoracic epidural catheterization. Anesthesiology 1997;86: 55–63.

36. Kang XH, Bao FP, Xiong XX, et al. Major complications of epidural anesthesia: a prospective study of 5083 cases at a single hospital. Acta Anaesthesiol Scand 2014;58:858–66.

37. Suksompong S, Pongpayuha P, Lertpaitoonpan W, et al. Low-dose spinal morphine for post-thoracotomy pain: a prospective randomized study. J Cardiothorac Vasc Anesth 2013;27:417–22.

38. Aun C, Thomas D, St John-Jones L, et al. Intrathecal morphine in cardiac surgery. Eur J Anaesthesiol 1985;2:419–26.

39. Roediger L, Joris J, Senard M, et al. The use of pre-operative intrathecal morphine for analgesia following coronary artery bypass surgery. Anaesthesia 2006;61:838–44.

40. Lena P, Balarac N, Arnulf JJ, et al. Intrathecal morphine and clonidine for coronary artery bypass grafting. Br J Anaesth 2003;90:300–3.

41. Etches RC. Respiratory depression associated with patient-controlled analgesia: a review of eight cases. Can J Anaesth 1994;41:125–32.

42. Ouerghi S, Fnaeich F, Frikha N, et al. The effect of adding intrathecal magnesium sulphate to morphine-fentanyl spinal analgesia after thoracic surgery. A prospective, double-blind, placebo-controlled research study. Ann Fr Anesth Reanim 2011;30:25–30.

43. Gwirtz KH, Young JV, Byers RS, et al. The safety and efficacy of intrathecal opioid analgesia for acute postoperative pain: seven years' experience with 5969 surgical patients at Indiana University Hospital. Anesth Analg 1999;88:599–604.

44. Dango S, Harris S, Offner K, et al. Combined paravertebral and intrathecal vs thoracic epidural analgesia for post-thoracotomy pain relief. Br J Anaesth 2013;110:443–9.

45. Madi-Jebara S, Adaimé C, Yazigi A, et al. Thoracic epidural and intrathecal analgesia have similar effects on pain relief and respiratory function after thoracic surgery. Can J Anaesth 2005; 52:710–6.

46. Piccioni F, Langer M, Fumagalli L, et al. Thoracic paravertebral anaesthesia for awake video-assisted thoracoscopic surgery daily. Anaesthesia 2010;65:1221–4.

47. Rusch VW, Mountain C. Thoracoscopy under regional anesthesia for the diagnosis and management of pleural disease. Am J Surg 1987;154: 274–8.

48. Dong Q, Liang L, Li Y, et al. Anesthesia with nontracheal intubation in thoracic surgery. J Thorac Dis 2012;4:126–30.

49. Migliore M, Giuliano R, Aziz T, et al. Four-step local anesthesia and sedation for thoracoscopic diagnosis and management of pleural diseases. Chest 2002;121:2032–5.

50. Katlic MR, Facktor MA. Video-assisted thoracic surgery utilizing local anesthesia and sedation: 384 consecutive cases. Ann Thorac Surg 2010;90: 240–5.

51. Adhikary SD, Pruett A, Forero M, et al. Erector spinae plane block as an alternative to epidural analgesia for post-operative analgesia following video-assisted thoracoscopic surgery: a case study and a literature review on the spread of local anaesthetic in the erector spinae plane. Indian J Anaesth 2018; 62:75–8.

52. Hernandez MA, Palazzi L, Lapalma J, et al. Erector spinae plane block for surgery of the posterior thoracic wall in a pediatric patient. Reg Anesth Pain Med 2018;43:217–9.

53. Yamak Altinpulluk E, García Simón D, Fajardo-Pérez M. Erector spinae plane block for analgesia after lower segment caesarean section: case report. Rev Esp Anestesiol Reanim 2018;65(5): 284–6.

54. Sullivan TR, Kanda P, Gagne S, et al. Harlequin syndrome associated with erector spinae plane block. Anesthesiology 2019. https://doi.org/10.1097/ALN. 0000000000002733.

55. Roy M. Pectoral block proven effective as motor block, but not skin sensory block. Annual meeting of the Canadian Anesthesiologists' Society, 2018. (abstract 446640).

56. Corso RM, Maitan S, Russotto V, et al. Type I and II pectoral nerve blocks with serratus plane block for awake video-assisted thoracic surgery. Anaesth Intensive Care 2016;44:643–4.

57. Chaudhri BB, Macfie A, Kirk AJ. Inadvertent total spinal anaesthesia after intercostal nerve block placement during lung resection. Ann Thorac Surg 2009;88:283–4.

58. Bello M, Oger S, Bedon-Carte S, et al. Effect of opioid-free anaesthesia on postoperative epidural ropivacaine requirement after thoracic surgery: a retrospective unmatched case-control study. Anaesth Crit Care Pain Med 2019. https://doi.org/ 10.1016/j.accpm.2019.01.013.

59. Guarracino F, Gemignani R, Pratesi G, et al. Awake palliative thoracic surgery in a high-risk patient: one-lung, non-invasive ventilation combined with epidural blockade. Anaesthesia 2008;63:761–3.

60. Guo Z, Shao W, Yin W, et al. Analysis of feasibility and safety of complete video-assisted thoracoscopic resection of anatomic pulmonary segments under non-intubated anesthesia. J Thorac Dis 2014;6:37–44.
61. Iwata Y, Hamai Y, Koyama T. Anesthetic management of nonintubated video-assisted thoracoscopic surgery using epidural anesthesia and dexmedetomidine in three patients with severe respiratory dysfunction. J Anesth 2016;30:324–7.
62. Bunch TJ, Ellenbogen KA, Packer DL, et al. Vagus nerve injury after posterior atrial radiofrequency ablation. Heart Rhythm 2008;5:1327–30.
63. Goel V, Patwardhan AM, Ibrahim M, et al. Complications associated with stellate ganglion nerve block: a systematic review. Reg Anesth Pain Med 2019. https://doi.org/10.1136/rapm-2018-100127.
64. Honda H, Honma T, Baba H. Epidural anesthesia with noninvasive positive pressure ventilation in a patient with compromised respiratory function. Masui 2010;59:467–9.
65. Hung MH, Hsu HH, Chan KC, et al. Non-intubated thoracoscopic surgery using internal intercostal nerve block, vagal block and targeted sedation. Eur J Cardiothorac Surg 2014;46:620–5.
66. McKenna RJ Jr. Lobectomy by video-assisted thoracic surgery with mediastinal node sampling for lung cancer. J Thorac Cardiovasc Surg 1994;107:879–81.
67. Green SM, Clem KJ, Rothrock SG. Ketamine safety profile in the developing world: survey of practitioners. Acad Emerg Med 1996;3:598–604.
68. Lodenius Å, Ebberyd A, Hårdemark Cedborg A, et al. Sedation with dexmedetomidine or propofol impairs hypoxic control of breathing in healthy male volunteers: a nonblinded, randomized crossover study. Anesthesiology 2016;125:700–15.
69. Ueshima H, Otake H. Emergency insertion of the LMA protector airway in patients in the lateral position. J Clin Anesth 2018;44:116.
70. Milling LS. Is high hypnotic suggestibility necessary for successful hypnotic pain intervention? Curr Pain Headache Rep 2008;12:98–102.
71. Barber J. Rapid induction analgesia: a clinical report. Am J Clin Hypn 1977;19:138–45.
72. Knoll H, Ziegeler S, Schreiber JU, et al. Airway injuries after one-lung ventilation: a comparison between double-lumen tube and endobronchial blocker: a randomized, prospective, controlled trial. Anesthesiology 2006;105:471–7.
73. Facco E, Pasquali S, Zanette G, et al. Hypnosis as sole anaesthesia for skin tumour removal in a patient with multiple chemical sensitivity. Anaesthesia 2013;68:961–5.
74. Kiss G, Butler J. Hypnosis for cataract surgery in an American Society of Anesthesiologists physical status IV patient. Anaesth Intensive Care 2011;39:1139–41.
75. Benumof JL. Chapter 2: distribution of ventilation and perfusion. In: Benumof JL, editor. Anesthesia for thoracic surgery. 2nd edition. Philadelphia: WB Saunders; 1995. p. 35–52.
76. Katlic MR. Video-assisted thoracic surgery utilizing local anesthesia and sedation. Eur J Cardiothorac Surg 2006;30:529–32.
77. Lan Lan AE, Jiayang Li BD, Xin Xu B, et al. Lung volume reduction under spontaneous ventilation in a patient with severe emphysema. Am J Case Rep 2019;20:125–30.
78. Gonzalez-Rivas D, Bonome C, Fieira E, et al. Nonintubated video-assisted thoracoscopic lung resections: the future of thoracic surgery? Eur J Cardiothorac Surg 2016;49:721–31.
79. Agzarian J, Shargall Y. Open thoracic surgery: video-assisted thoracoscopic surgery (VATS) conversion to thoracotomy. Shanghai Chest 2017;1:31.
80. Decaluwe H, Petersen RH, Hansen H, et al. Major intraoperative complications during video-assisted thoracoscopic anatomical lung resections: an intention-to-treat analysis. Eur J Cardiothorac Surg 2015;48:588–98.
81. Ovassapian A. Conduct of anesthesia. In: Shields TW, LoCicero J, Ponn RB, editors. General thoracic surgery. Philadelphia: Lippincott Williams & Wilkins; 2000. p. 327–44.
82. Liu J, Cui F, Li S, et al. Nonintubated video-assisted thoracoscopic surgery under epidural anesthesia compared with conventional anesthetic option: a randomized control study. Surg Innov 2015;22:123–30.
83. Kiss G, Castillo M. Nonintubated anesthesia in thoracic surgery: general issues. Ann Transl Med 2015;3:110.
84. Sunaga H, Blasberg JD, Heerdt PM. Anesthesia for nonintubated video-assisted thoracic surgery. Curr Opin Anaesthesiol 2017;30:1–6.
85. Macchiarini P, Rovira I, Ferrarello S. Awake upper airway surgery. Ann Thorac Surg 2010;89:387–90.
86. Irons JF, Martinez G. Anaesthetic considerations for non-intubated thoracic surgery. J Vis Surg 2016;2:61.
87. Frerk C, Mitchell VS, McNarry AF, et al, Difficult Airway Society Intubation Guidelines Working Group. Difficult Airway Society 2015 guidelines for management of unanticipated difficult intubation in adults. Br J Anaesth 2015;115:827–48.
88. Brodsky JB. Lung separation and the difficult airway. Br J Anaesth 2009;103(Suppl 1):i66–75.
89. Rim SK, Son YB, Kim JI, et al. Propofol and remifentanil total intravenous anesthesia and the

preservation of spontaneous respiration for a patient with mediastinal mass. Korean J Anesthesiol 2013; 65:583–4.

90. Takara I, Uehara M, Higa Y, et al. Respiratory management in a patient with severe tracheal stenosis caused by compression from the ascending aortic arch aneurysm. Masui 2003;52:1079–82 [in Japanese].

91. Hattamer SJ, Dodds TM. Use of the laryngeal mask airway in managing a patient with a large anterior mediastinal mass: a case report. AANA J 1996;64: 497–500.

Nonintubated Video-Assisted Thoracic Surgery for the Management of Primary and Secondary Spontaneous Pneumothorax

Pei-Hsing Chen, MD[a], Wan-Ting Hung, MD[b], Jin-Shing Chen, MD, PhD[c],*

KEYWORDS

- Thoracoscopic surgery • Pneumothorax • Video-assisted thoracic surgery • Bullectomy

KEY POINTS

- Nonintubated video-assisted thoracoscopic surgery (VATS) is a feasible and safe alternative for the management of primary or secondary spontaneous pneumothorax.
- A variety of anesthetic techniques have been reported, and methods for managing the airway, analgesia, and sedation should be separately considered.
- Surgical techniques for nonintubated VATS bullectomy and pleurodesis are similar to those for the intubated approach.
- Hypercapnia may become intolerant in risky patients, and noninvasive ventilator should be prepared.

INTRODUCTION

Definition

The term pneumothorax was first presented in 1803. At that time, most cases of pneumothorax were secondary to tuberculosis, although some involved otherwise healthy patients ("pneumothorax simple"). The term "primary spontaneous pneumothorax" (PSP) was first used in 1932 to describe pneumothorax in healthy young individuals with no underlying respiratory disease. Currently, pneumothorax is classified by the cause or according to the underlying respiratory disease. PSP is defined as pneumothorax without traumatic injury or related pulmonary disease, whereas secondary spontaneous pneumothorax (SSP) refers to pneumothorax that develops in the presence of an underlying pulmonary condition, such as chronic obstructive pulmonary disease (COPD), cystic fibrosis, or *Pneumocystis carinii* pneumonia. Because of the effect of the preexisting lung disease, the management of SSP is potentially more difficult.

Treatment Choice and Indications

Currently, the optimal treatment of PSP and SSP is debatable. Generally, observation, simple aspiration, and chest tube insertion are used in the initial treatment course, whereas surgery and

Disclosure Statement: The authors have nothing to disclose.
[a] Division of Thoracic Surgery, Department of Surgery, National Taiwan University Hospital Yun-Lin Branch, No. 579, Sec. 2, Yun-Lin Road, Douliu City, Yun-Lin County 64041, Taiwan; [b] Division of Thoracic Surgery, Department of Surgery, National Taiwan University Hospital, No. 7, Chung-Shan South Road, Taipei 10002, Taiwan; [c] Division of Thoracic Surgery, Department of Surgery, National Taiwan University Hospital, National Taiwan University College of Medicine, No. 7, Chung-Shan South Road, Taipei 10002, Taiwan
* Corresponding author.
E-mail address: chenjs@ntu.edu.tw

pleurodesis are suggested for recurrent or complicated pneumothorax.[1,2] Surgical intervention involving video-assisted thoracic surgery (VATS) for bullectomy and pleurodesis (**Fig. 1**) has shown satisfactory results, with most procedures performed under general anesthesia with lung isolation using a double-lumen endotracheal tube.[3]

Double-lumen endobronchial tubes have been used since the development of modern thoracic surgery in 1959. These tubes facilitate single-lung ventilation, are safe, and allow easy manipulation of the lungs.[4] However, several unavoidable disadvantages have been recorded over decades of observation; these include postoperative pneumonia, impaired cardiopulmonary function, ventilator-related barotrauma, lung atelectasis in both dependent and nondependent individuals, neuromuscular side effects, and major airway injury.[4–6] Fortunately, rapid improvements in minimally invasive surgeries, primarily VATS, have resulted in the development and evolution of nonintubation anesthesia, with several studies proving its safety and feasibility in cases involving various thoracic conditions, such as solitary lung tumors (resection),[6–16] interstitial disease, empyema thoracis (pleural decortication),[17] mediastinal tumors (excision),[18–20] bullous disease associated with pneumothorax,[21–28] and emphysematous pulmonary disease.[29–35] The aim of the present review is to discuss the feasibility and outcomes of nonintubated thoracoscopic surgery for pneumothorax.

FACTORS INVOLVED IN NONINTUBATED VIDEO-ASSISTED THORACOSCOPIC SURGERY
Respiratory Physiology: Oxygenation and Ventilation

For the maintenance of an effortless respiratory pattern during surgery, there should be no obvious mismatch between the alveolar ventilation (V) and alveolar blood flow/perfusion (Q), particularly in patients with compromised cardiopulmonary function. Conditions with a mismatch between ventilation and perfusion (V/Q mismatch), such as heart failure, pulmonary embolism, lung collapse, and sputum accumulation, which exhibit a high incidence in older patients with chronic cardiopulmonary diseases (COPD, interstitial lung disease [ILD], cystic fibrosis), can compromise the efficiency of oxygenation.

Locoregional Anesthesia

Generally, the area of regional anesthesia includes the chest cage and parietal pleura. Commonly used techniques include thoracic epidural anesthesia/analgesia (TEA), paravertebral nerve block, percutaneous or thoracoscopic intercostal nerve block (ICNB), and intrapleural analgesia. However, each technique has certain indications and contraindications, particularly for high-risk patients.

TEA can also induce motor blockade in the respiratory muscles within the thoracic cage, with a 10% decline in the lung volume (vital capacity, functional residual capacity [FRC], forced vital capacity [FVC], and forced expiratory volume in 1 second [FEV1]).[5,36] Moreover, it is a time-consuming and technically demanding procedure and can cause peripheral vasodilation and functional hypovolemia owing to sympathetic blockade.[37] Neurologic and cardiorespiratory complications have also been occasionally reported.[38] Consequently, ICNB is sometimes used as an alternative. Vagus nerve block and intravenous narcotics are also reliable tools for minimizing visceral pain.[7,8,11,13–16,39–44] These methods preserve the phrenic nerve (origin in the neck [C3 to C5]), consequently maintaining the function of the diaphragm.

Anesthetic Management

With regard to the sedation level during nonintubated VATS, patients are generally fully awake or moderately to deeply sedated. Diverse depths of sedation are particularly necessary for anxious patients or patients requiring prolonged surgery. Inhaled anesthetics administered through laryngeal airway masks and intravenous anesthetics (eg, propofol, midazolam) (**Fig. 2**) have shown satisfactory results in such cases,[38,45,46] although these anesthetic agents inadvertently reduce FRC.[47]

Spontaneous Breathing

Preservation of FRC of the dependent lung is one of the benefits of nonintubated surgery. In intubated patients, the overall FRC reduces once the

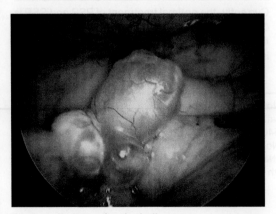
Fig. 1. Bulla lesion for the bullectomy.

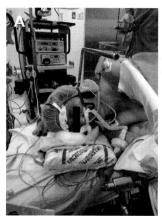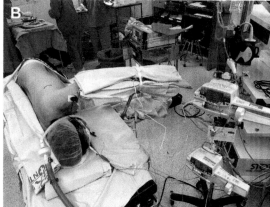

Fig. 2. (A) Anesthetic settings of nonintubated VATS. (B) Overview of anesthetic settings.

induction of anesthesia is initiated. As a result, the nondependent lung becomes more compliant, whereas the dependent lung shifts to a less compliant area in the pulmonary compliance curve.[48] Administration of a muscle relaxant for ventilation control results in redirection of the tidal volume. Without spontaneous diaphragmatic contraction, the abdominal pressure results in increased tension and, consequently, an obvious reduction in FRC.[47,49]

Permissive Hypercapnia

Without lung separation, communication between the dependent and nondependent lungs during surgical pneumothorax would lead to "carbon dioxide rebreathing," which results in hypercapnia.[50] Because the hypercapnia can trigger tachypnea, respiratory depressants, such as opioids or sedatives, are administered in these cases. In the past, respiratory depressants were associated with concerns about deterioration in ventilation and oxygenation. However, more recent studies have shown that the degree of hypoventilation induced by these agents is not clinically significant.[4,13,51] A face mask, a laryngeal mask airway, a high-flow nasal cannula, or an oropharyngeal cannula can be used for supplemental oxygen delivery.[7,11,12,52,53] A perioperative increase in the carbon dioxide level is not considered harmful if it is within the range used for permissive hypercapnia.[4,13,51]

Surgical Pneumothorax

Surgical pneumothorax is created after opening the nondependent hemithorax. The dependent lung would bear the full weight of the mediastinum because of the lack of a negative intrapleural pressure in the nondependent hemithorax. At this time, reductions in FRC and the ventilation volume

become apparent.[50] Moreover, there is a decrease in the caval venous return, which results in a decrease in the cardiac output and pulmonary perfusion.[54] The increasing vascular resistance in the collapsed nondependent lung may shift the pulmonary blood to the dependent lung and improve the V/Q ratio. Nevertheless, the decline in the cardiac output may worsen the blood oxygen-carrying capacity, influence the mixed oxygen saturation, and deteriorate oxygenation.[54,55] The use of a sedative drug or TEA can significantly influence this compensation. The medication should be carefully titrated, particularly for patients with impaired cardiopulmonary function.[56,57]

RATIONALE AND POTENTIAL ADVANTAGES OF NONINTUBATED VIDEO-ASSISTED THORACOSCOPIC SURGERY FOR SPONTANEOUS PNEUMOTHORAX
Primary Spontaneous Pneumothorax

Patients with PSP are mostly young adults without contraindications for nonintubated VATS. In the field of minimally invasive thoracic surgery, nonintubated VATS is potentially a less invasive procedure for the management of PSP[22,23] and is associated with better procedure acceptance, faster postoperative recovery, and a shorter hospital stay. Furthermore, surgery-related costs may decrease because of the low incidence of adverse effects.[27]

Secondary Spontaneous pneumothorax

Patients with SSP are generally elderly with an underlying pleural or pulmonary disease, namely COPD, ILD, or cystic fibrosis or other less common diseases. Regardless of the cause, the morbidities and mortalities for SSP are higher than those for PSP. In most patients with SSP, the performance status and cardiopulmonary function are generally poor, with a high likelihood of a reduced FEV1 and FEV1/FVC ratio.[2,29]

General anesthesia in SSP patients can result in hemodynamic instability, alveolar barotrauma, volutrauma, and atelectrauma in the perioperative period, and some patients cannot undergo surgery because of the impaired pulmonary function and high incidence of cardiopulmonary complications caused by general anesthesia. Therefore, conservative treatment has often been the first line of treatment in the past. However, of late, the role of surgical treatment, particularly VATS, has become indisputable. Although most VATS procedures for SSP are performed under general anesthesia, nonintubated VATS precludes the need for general anesthesia and prevents ventilator-induced damage. Previous reports recommend that patients with SSP who are contraindicated for surgery because of the risk of cardiopulmonary complications should undergo awake surgery performed by experienced surgeons.[28] Studies by Noda and colleagues[33] and Mineo and Ambrogi[31] also showed the clinical benefits of awake thoracoscopic surgery in patients with SSP, including a lower incidence of postoperative respiratory complications and reduced expression of stress hormones and systemic inflammatory markers. Avoidance of neuromuscular blockade, which prevents atelectasis in the nonoperated dependent lung and lowers the risk of hypoxia and ventilator dependency, is another important consideration in nonintubated surgery.[58] It maintains FRC and preserves the compliance of the dependent lung, thus maintaining adequate perfusion and preventing a V/Q mismatch. All of these effects are vital for patients with SSP. The risk of hypoxemia and hypercapnia is also lower with nonintubated anesthesia than with intubated general anesthesia.[59]

Previous research has documented the mechanism of hypoxic pulmonary vasoconstriction. The vessels in nonventilated areas are redirected to the ventilated areas. The volatile anesthetics used for general anesthesia suppress the compensation mechanism, whereas intravenous anesthetics, such as propofol, and TEA agents, such as bupivacaine, ropivacaine, and xylocaine, have a negligible influence on the mechanism of hypoxic pulmonary vasoconstriction.[60,61] Nonintubated surgery may be a safer choice for patients with long-term hypoxic conditions, such as pulmonary fibrosis and emphysema. Some metaanalyses showed that nonintubated surgery reduced cardiac morbidity and mortality after noncardiac procedures,[62,63] whereas other studies showed that nonintubated surgery could prevent a third of the pulmonary infections and half of the pulmonary complications induced by general anesthesia.[64] Nonintubated surgery is also associated with earlier mobilization and improved coughing ability because of lesser opioid use, which prevents the accumulation of secretions and prevents respiratory infection. These benefits lower the overall risk for patients with SSP.

ANESTHETIC CONSIDERATIONS
Anesthetic Choice

In 1997, Nezu and colleagues[28] reported the potential of local anesthesia (LA) with sedation during thoracic surgery for spontaneous pneumothorax. Subsequently, clinicians began using TEA, which became the most common analgesic technique (**Table 1**). TEA has been applied in almost every study concerning nonintubated thoracoscopic surgery for PSP and SSP. However, it is technically demanding and causes potential side effects; therefore, ICNB is used as an alternative technique for regional anesthesia. Guo and colleagues[65] reported a retrospective cohort study involving 240 cases subjected to VATS bullectomy under total intravenous anesthesia (TIVA)/TEA or TIVA/LA. The short-term outcomes and recurrence rates showed no significant differences between the 2 anesthetic techniques, and the investigators suggested that TIVA/LA may be a suitable alternative to TIVA/TEA for the surgical management of PSP.

Although intrathoracic vagal nerve block, which was described by Chen and colleagues,[13] can effectively inhibit the cough reflex during nonintubated VATS lobectomy,[7,8] only 1 study has used this technique in a cohort of patients with spontaneous pneumothorax.[25] This is probably because bullectomy and pleurodesis are minor procedures when compared with lobectomy, which involves dissection of the hilum. Furthermore, there are concerns about residual vagal nerve blockade (>3 hours), which can inhibit the cough reflex after surgery.

Hypercapnia

In nonintubated VATS, hypercapnia within a safe range, known as permissive hypercapnia, is a common phenomenon. Although it shows no obvious influence in patients with PSP, it may pose a problem in patients with SSP, particularly those with COPD. Patients with SSP may already exhibit chronic hypercapnia, and their carbon dioxide level can increase rapidly during surgery. Invasive arterial blood pressure monitoring is necessary in these patients. In addition, the level of sedation and opioid dose should be very carefully titrated. Inoue and colleagues[66] used

Table 1
Awake and nonintubated video-assisted thoracoscopic surgery performed for the treatment of primary spontaneous pneumothorax in different studies

First Author, y	Study Design	Patient Number	Anesthesia	Ports	Pleurodesis	Morbidity (%)	Recurrence Rate (%)	Hospital Stay
Nezu[a] et al,[28] 1997	Observational study	32	ICNB + TIVA	3	Fibrin glue	9.4	3.1	4.5 ± 1.3
Pompeo et al,[27] 2007	Randomized controlled trial	43	TEA/GA	3	Abrasion	4.5	4.5	2.0 ± 1.0
Rocco et al,[26] 2011	Case report	1	TEA + TIVA	1	Abrasion with talc pleurodesis	—	No	1[b,c]
Onodera et al,[24] 2013	Case report	1	TEA + TIVA	1[a]	—	—	No	2[b]
Chen et al,[1] 2013	Case report	1	TEA + TIVA + Vagal block	—	Abrasion	—	No	4[b]
Li et al,[23] 2015	Observational study	32	TEA + TIVA	1	—	—	0	1.7 ± 0.3
Guo et al,[65] 2016	Observational study	240	TIVA-TEA/TIVA-ICNB	2	—	2/2	3/2	3.4 ± 1.5/2.7 ± 1.5[b]

Abbreviations: —, not mentioned; GA, general anesthesia.
[a] PSP group + SSP group.
[b] Plus 2 needles.
[c] Postoperative hospital stay.

remifentanil, a titratable opioid with quick onset and washout, in order to slow the respiratory rate during bulla resection in a patient with acute respiratory failure. They found that the respiratory rate decreased to 6/minute, with rapid recovery within 1 minute after the remifentanil bolus. However, in cases of severe hypercapnia, a noninvasive ventilator should be prepared, and the sedative dose should be as low as possible.[29]

SURGICAL CONSIDERATIONS

There are no significant differences between intubated and nonintubated surgery for PSP and SSP in terms of the standard procedures and maneuvers. The primary goals are resection of the bullae and sealing of leak points. Unexpectedly, however, very few studies involving patients with PSP[25–27] and none involving patients with SSP used abrasion pleurodesis. Apical pleurectomy with talc pleurodesis is also used as per recommendations of the Respiratory Pathology Spanish Society,[67] American College of Chest Physicians,[3] and British Thoracic Society guidelines[2] (see **Table 1**), and the use of polyglycolic acid (PGA) sheets with fibrin glue is a more favorable option for SSP treated by nonintubated VATS (**Table 2**). Nonintubated single-access (uniportal) thoracoscopic surgery has also been reported for the management of PSP.[23]

FEASIBILITY AND OUTCOME
Patient Selection

Common contraindications for nonintubated VATS include an American Society of Anesthesiologists performance status of 3 to 5, bleeding disorders, sleep apnea, high risk of gastric reflux, a body mass index of greater than 30, and unstable asthma. It is also contraindicated in patients with expected severe pleural adhesions, which are more common in patients with SSP. Surgeries under general anesthesia for pneumothorax in patients with cardiopulmonary dysfunction are generally considered challenging, and it might be difficult to maintain adequate oxygenation during intubation and the postoperative course. However, previous reports have shown that nonintubated thoracoscopic surgery is feasible for high-risk patients with pneumothorax, including those with bilateral pneumothorax[26] or pneumoconiosis[35] and those who have undergone bone marrow transplantation,[32] single-lung transplantation,[34] or pneumonectomy.[33]

The optimal treatment of pneumothorax in pregnancy is debatable. General anesthesia during pregnancy can pose maternal and fetal risks, including teratogenicity and abortion. Therefore, it is better to avoid surgical intervention under general anesthesia in these patients. Nevertheless, sporadic case reports have demonstrated the applicability of awake or nonintubated VATS with satisfactory outcomes in pregnant patients with spontaneous pneumothorax.[24,25]

Perioperative Recovery and Recurrence

Although nonintubated thoracic surgery is considered to result in better recovery, the perioperative outcomes of nonintubated thoracoscopic surgery for spontaneous pneumothorax remain controversial. Nezu and colleagues[28] reported that nonintubated thoracoscopic surgery for spontaneous pneumothorax (PSP group and SSP group) required less time than did surgery under general anesthesia. However, a study by Pompeo and colleagues[27] could not confirm this finding in patients with PSP. A metaanalysis by Chen and colleagues[68] reported no significant differences between nonintubated anesthesia (including PSP and SSP groups) and general anesthesia groups in terms of the surgical duration, length of hospital stay, and complication rate. Overall, studies on nonintubated thoracoscopic surgery are very few, with no clinical trial performed to verify the perioperative outcomes of this procedure in patients with SSP.

Recognition of blebs or bullae is considered the most important step of surgery for spontaneous pneumothorax, because it not only affects the surgical duration but also determines the recurrence rate. Some critics state that the nonintubated method may increase the difficulty in identifying the bullae, thus prolonging the procedure and increasing the recurrence rate. However, Guo and colleagues[65] showed no difference in the recurrence rate between surgery under TIVA/LA (2%) or TIVA/TEA (3%) and surgery under general anesthesia (5%) in patients with PSP. In addition, Pompeo and colleagues[27] reported no differences in the intraoperative detection rate for emphysema-like changes between nonintubated VATS and surgery under general anesthesia in patients with PSP (90% vs 95%; $P = .52$). In fact, Nezu and colleagues[28] mentioned that the nonintubated approach can even assist in the detection of small blebs/bullae that remain inflated during spontaneous breathing. Although further evidence is necessary, current available studies show that the nonintubated method allows good exposure and adequate resection of the affected areas in patients with PSP. In general, the reported recurrence rates after nonintubated thoracoscopic surgery for PSP or SSP are satisfactory (see **Tables**

Table 2
Awake and nonintubated video-assisted thoracoscopic surgery performed for the treatment of secondary spontaneous pneumothorax in different studies

First Author, y	Study Design	Number	Anesthesia	Ports	Pleurodesis	Morbidity (%)	Recurrence Rate (%)	Hospital Stay
Nezu[a] et al,[28] 1997	Observational study	32	ICNB + TIVA	3	Fibrin glue	9.4	3.2	4.5 ± 1.3
Tschopp,[70] 1997	Observational study	93	ICNB + TIVA	2	Talc pleurodesis	6.4	6.4	5.2
Mukaida et al,[35] 1998	Observational study	4	TEA + ICNB + TIVA	3	PGA sheet + fibrin glue	0	0	5[b]
Sugimoto et al,[34] 2005	Case report	2	TEA + ICNB	3	PGA sheet	—	No	—
Inoue et al,[66] 2010	Case report	1	TEA	—	—	—	No	
Shigematsu et al,[32] 2011	Case report	1	TEA + ICNB	—	PGA sheet + fibrin glue	—	No	
Noda et al,[33] 2011	Case report	1	TEA + ICNB	2	PGA sheet + fibrin glue	—	No	4[c]
Noda et al,[30] 2012	Observational study	15	TEA + ICNB	3	PGA sheet + fibrin glue	26.7	—	26.3 ± 33.8
Ahn et al,[67] 2017	Observational study	33	TEA ± ICNB	2 or 3	Neoveil ± talc pleurodesis	3 (1[b])	3	7.97 ± 5.43

[a] PSP group + SSP group.
[b] Postoperative chest drainage.
[c] Postoperative hospital stay.

1 and **2**). Even though surgical mortality has been reported in high-risk patients,[69] this method is considered a safe and reliable alternative for the management of PSP and SSP. Currently, no study has documented cases of conversion; however, a noninvasive ventilator should be prepared under consideration of possible hypercapnia beyond the permissible range.

LIMITATIONS

Since the first report of nonintubated VATS for spontaneous pneumothorax was published by Nezu and colleagues,[28] several studies have attempted to establish the feasibility and safety of this method. Even then, evidence of its benefits is not strong enough, with the complete lack of clinical trials involving patients with SSP. Moreover, after Mineo and Ambrogi[31] described the possible role of stress hormones and biomarkers of systemic inflammation in the outcomes of nonintubated thoracoscopic surgery in 2012, no further studies have evaluated the immune response, which may be related to the occurrence of postoperative complications. In addition, considering the diversity of anesthetic techniques and surgical choices, the optimal combination remains unknown.

SUMMARY

Nonintubated thoracoscopic surgery for spontaneous pneumothorax is a feasible and safe alternative for patients with persistent or recurrent pneumothorax. Research in the past 20 years has focused on the perioperative outcomes, including the surgical duration, length of hospital stay, and postoperative morbidity and respiratory complication rates, which appear to be better than those of surgery under general anesthesia. This technique is also a suitable alternative for patients who cannot receive general anesthesia because of increased risks. Further randomized trials are necessary to confirm these benefits.

REFERENCES

1. Chen JS, Chan WK, Tsai KT, et al. Simple aspiration and drainage and intrapleural minocycline pleurodesis versus simple aspiration and drainage for the initial treatment of primary spontaneous pneumothorax: an open-label, parallel-group, prospective, randomised, controlled trial. Lancet 2013;381:1277–82.
2. MacDuff A, Arnold A, Harvey J. Management of spontaneous pneumothorax: British Thoracic Society Pleural Disease Guideline 2010. Thorax 2010;65(Suppl 2):ii18–31.
3. Baumann MH, Strange C, Heffner JE, et al. Management of spontaneous pneumothorax: an American College of Chest Physicians Delphi consensus statement. Chest 2001;119:590–602.
4. Pompeo E. State of the art and perspectives in nonintubated thoracic surgery. Ann Transl Med 2014;2:106.
5. Groeben H. Epidural anesthesia and pulmonary function. J Anesth 2006;20:290–9.
6. Hung MH, Hsu HH, Cheng YJ, et al. Nonintubated thoracoscopic surgery: state of the art and future directions. J Thorac Dis 2014;6:2–9.
7. Wang ML, Hung MH, Hsu HH, et al. Non-intubated thoracoscopic surgery for lung cancer in patients with impaired pulmonary function. Ann Transl Med 2019;7:40.
8. Hung WT, Hung MH, Wang ML, et al. Nonintubated thoracoscopic surgery for lung tumor: seven years' experience with 1,025 patients. Ann Thorac Surg 2019;107:1607–12.
9. Wang ML, Galvez C, Chen JS, et al. Non-intubated single-incision video-assisted thoracic surgery: a two-center cohort of 188 patients. J Thorac Dis 2017;9:2587–98.
10. Gonzalez-Rivas D. Uniportal thoracoscopic surgery: from medical thoracoscopy to non-intubated uniportal video-assisted major pulmonary resections. Ann Cardiothorac Surg 2016;5:85–91.
11. Chen JS, Cheng YJ, Hung MH, et al. Nonintubated thoracoscopic lobectomy for lung cancer. Ann Surg 2011;254:1038–43.
12. Pompeo E, Mineo D, Rogliani P, et al. Feasibility and results of awake thoracoscopic resection of solitary pulmonary nodules. Ann Thorac Surg 2004;78:1761–8.
13. Chen KC, Cheng YJ, Hung MH, et al. Nonintubated thoracoscopic lung resection: a 3-year experience with 285 cases in a single institution. J Thorac Dis 2012;4:347–51.
14. Hung MH, Hsu HH, Chen KC, et al. Nonintubated thoracoscopic anatomical segmentectomy for lung tumors. Ann Thorac Surg 2013;96:1209–15.
15. Hung MH, Cheng YJ, Chan KC, et al. Nonintubated uniportal thoracoscopic surgery for peripheral lung nodules. Ann Thorac Surg 2014;98:1998–2003.
16. Hung MH, Cheng YJ, Hsu HH, et al. Nonintubated uniportal thoracoscopic segmentectomy for lung cancer. J Thorac Cardiovasc Surg 2014;148:e234–5.
17. Tacconi F, Pompeo E, Fabbi E, et al. Awake video-assisted pleural decortication for empyema thoracis. Eur J Cardiothorac Surg 2010;37:594–601.
18. Pompeo E, Tacconi F, Mineo TC. Awake video-assisted thoracoscopic biopsy in complex anterior

mediastinal masses. Thorac Surg Clin 2010;20: 225–33.

19. Matsumoto I, Oda M, Watanabe G. Awake endoscopic thymectomy via an infrasternal approach using sternal lifting. Thorac Cardiovasc Surg 2008;56: 311–3.

20. Tsunezuka Y, Oda M, Matsumoto I, et al. Extended thymectomy in patients with myasthenia gravis with high thoracic epidural anesthesia alone. World J Surg 2004;28:962–5 [discussion: 965–6].

21. Tsai TM, Lin MW, Li YJ, et al. The size of spontaneous pneumothorax is a predictor of unsuccessful catheter drainage. Sci Rep 2017;7:181.

22. Bertolaccini L, Pardolesi A, Brandolini J, et al. Uniportal video-assisted thoracic surgery for pneumothorax and blebs/bullae. J Vis Surg 2017;3:107.

23. Li S, Cui F, Liu J, et al. Nonintubated uniportal videoassisted thoracoscopic surgery for primary spontaneous pneumothorax. Chin J Cancer Res 2015;27: 197–202.

24. Onodera K, Noda M, Okada Y, et al. Awake videothoracoscopic surgery for intractable pneumothorax in pregnancy by using a single portal plus puncture. Interact Cardiovasc Thorac Surg 2013;17:438–40.

25. Chen YH, Hung MH, Chen JS, et al. Nonintubated video-assisted thoracoscopic surgery (VATS) for recurrent spontaneous pneumothorax in a pregnant woman: 11AP5-10. Eur J Anaesthesiol 2013;30:180.

26. Rocco G, La Rocca A, Martucci N, et al. Awake single-access (uniportal) video-assisted thoracoscopic surgery for spontaneous pneumothorax. J Thorac Cardiovasc Surg 2011;142:944–5.

27. Pompeo E, Tacconi F, Mineo D, et al. The role of awake video-assisted thoracoscopic surgery in spontaneous pneumothorax. J Thorac Cardiovasc Surg 2007;133:786–90.

28. Nezu K, Kushibe K, Tojo T, et al. Thoracoscopic wedge resection of blebs under local anesthesia with sedation for treatment of a spontaneous pneumothorax. Chest 1997;111:230–5.

29. Galvez C, Bolufer S, Navarro-Martinez J, et al. Nonintubated video-assisted thoracic surgery management of secondary spontaneous pneumothorax. Ann Transl Med 2015;3:104.

30. Noda M, Okada Y, Maeda S, et al. Is there a benefit of awake thoracoscopic surgery in patients with secondary spontaneous pneumothorax? J Thorac Cardiovasc Surg 2012;143:613–6.

31. Mineo TC, Ambrogi V. Awake thoracic surgery for secondary spontaneous pneumothorax: another advancement. J Thorac Cardiovasc Surg 2012; 144:1533–4.

32. Shigematsu H, Andou A, Matsuo K, et al. Thoracoscopic surgery using local and epidural anesthesia for intractable pneumothorax after BMT. Bone Marrow Transplant 2011;46:472–3.

33. Noda M, Okada Y, Maeda S, et al. Successful thoracoscopic surgery for intractable pneumothorax after pneumonectomy under local and epidural anesthesia. J Thorac Cardiovasc Surg 2011;141: 1545–7.

34. Sugimoto S, Date H, Sugimoto R, et al. Thoracoscopic operation with local and epidural anesthesia in the treatment of pneumothorax after lung transplantation. J Thorac Cardiovasc Surg 2005;130: 1219–20.

35. Mukaida T, Andou A, Date H, et al. Thoracoscopic operation for secondary pneumothorax under local and epidural anesthesia in high-risk patients. Ann Thorac Surg 1998;65:924–6.

36. Warner DO, Warner MA, Ritman EL. Human chest wall function during epidural anesthesia. Anesthesiology 1996;85:761–73.

37. Clemente A, Carli F. The physiological effects of thoracic epidural anesthesia and analgesia on the cardiovascular, respiratory and gastrointestinal systems. Minerva Anestesiol 2008;74:549–63.

38. Hung MH, Hsu HH, Chan KC, et al. Non-intubated thoracoscopic surgery using internal intercostal nerve block, vagal block and targeted sedation. Eur J Cardiothorac Surg 2014;46:620–5.

39. Hung MH, Chen JS, Cheng YJ. Precise anesthesia in thoracoscopic operations. Curr Opin Anaesthesiol 2019;32:39–43.

40. Yang SM, Wang ML, Hung MH, et al. Tubeless uniportal thoracoscopic wedge resection for peripheral lung nodules. Ann Thorac Surg 2017;103: 462–8.

41. Tsai TM, Lin MW, Hsu HH, et al. Nonintubated uniportal thoracoscopic wedge resection for early lung cancer. J Vis Surg 2017;3:155.

42. Hung MH, Yang SM, Chen JS. Nonintubated videoassisted thoracic surgery lobectomy for lung cancer. J Vis Surg 2017;3:10.

43. Hung WT, Liao HC, Cheng YJ, et al. Nonintubated thoracoscopic pneumonectomy for bullous emphysema. Ann Thorac Surg 2016;102:e353–5.

44. Wu CY, Chen JS, Lin YS, et al. Feasibility and safety of nonintubated thoracoscopic lobectomy for geriatric lung cancer patients. Ann Thorac Surg 2013; 95:405–11.

45. Mineo TC. Epidural anesthesia in awake thoracic surgery. Eur J Cardiothorac Surg 2007;32:13–9.

46. Liu J, Cui F, Li S, et al. Nonintubated video-assisted thoracoscopic surgery under epidural anesthesia compared with conventional anesthetic option: a randomized control study. Surg Innov 2015;22: 123–30.

47. Hedenstierna G, Edmark L. The effects of anesthesia and muscle paralysis on the respiratory system. Intensive Care Med 2005;31:1327–35.

48. Wahba RW. Perioperative functional residual capacity. Can J Anaesth 1991;38:384–400.

49. Lohser JIS. Physiology of the lateral decubitus position, open chest and one-lung ventilation. In: Slinger P, editor. Principles and practice of anesthesia for thoracic surgery. New York: Springer Science; 2011. p. 71–82.

50. Pompeo E. Awake thoracic surgery–is it worth the trouble? Semin Thorac Cardiovasc Surg 2012;24:106–14.

51. Pompeo E, Rogliani P, Tacconi F, et al. Randomized comparison of awake nonresectional versus nonawake resectional lung volume reduction surgery. J Thorac Cardiovasc Surg 2012;143:47–54, 54.e1.

52. Galvez C, Navarro-Martinez J, Bolufer S, et al. Nonintubated uniportal VATS pulmonary anatomical resections. J Vis Surg 2017;3:120.

53. Ambrogi MC, Fanucchi O, Gemignani R, et al. Video-assisted thoracoscopic surgery with spontaneous breathing laryngeal mask anesthesia: preliminary experience. J Thorac Cardiovasc Surg 2012;144:514–5.

54. Li TH, Rheinlander HF, Etsten B. Circulatory changes due to open pneumothorax in surgical patients. Anesthesiology 1960;21:171–7.

55. Levin AI, Coetzee JF, Coetzee A. Arterial oxygenation and one-lung anesthesia. Curr Opin Anaesthesiol 2008;21:28–36.

56. Liu YJ, Hung MH, Hsu HH, et al. Effects on respiration of nonintubated anesthesia in thoracoscopic surgery under spontaneous ventilation. Ann Transl Med 2015;3:107.

57. Yang JT, Hung MH, Chen JS, et al. Anesthetic consideration for nonintubated VATS. J Thorac Dis 2014;6:10–3.

58. Kiss G, Claret A, Desbordes J, et al. Thoracic epidural anaesthesia for awake thoracic surgery in severely dyspnoeic patients excluded from general anaesthesia. Interact Cardiovasc Thorac Surg 2014;19:816–23.

59. Kao MC, Lan CH, Huang CJ. Anesthesia for awake video-assisted thoracic surgery. Acta Anaesthesiol Taiwan 2012;50:126–30.

60. Pruszkowski O, Dalibon N, Moutafis M, et al. Effects of propofol vs sevoflurane on arterial oxygenation during one-lung ventilation. Br J Anaesth 2007;98:539–44.

61. Nagendran J, Stewart K, Hoskinson M, et al. An anesthesiologist's guide to hypoxic pulmonary vasoconstriction: implications for managing single-lung anesthesia and atelectasis. Curr Opin Anaesthesiol 2006;19:34–43.

62. Beattie WS, Badner NH, Choi P. Epidural analgesia reduces postoperative myocardial infarction: a meta-analysis. Anesth Analg 2001;93:853–8.

63. Wijeysundera DN, Beattie WS, Austin PC, et al. Epidural anaesthesia and survival after intermediate-to-high risk non-cardiac surgery: a population-based cohort study. Lancet 2008;372:562–9.

64. Ballantyne JC, Carr DB, deFerranti S, et al. The comparative effects of postoperative analgesic therapies on pulmonary outcome: cumulative meta-analyses of randomized, controlled trials. Anesth Analg 1998;86:598–612.

65. Guo Z, Yin W, Wang W, et al. Spontaneous ventilation anaesthesia: total intravenous anaesthesia with local anaesthesia or thoracic epidural anaesthesia for thoracoscopic bullectomy. Eur J Cardiothorac Surg 2016;50:927–32.

66. Inoue K, Moriyama K, Takeda J. Remifentanil for awake thoracoscopic bullectomy. J Thorac Cardiovasc Surg 2010;24:386–7.

67. Rivas de Andres JJ, Jimenez Lopez MF, Molins Lopez-Rodo L, et al. Guidelines for the diagnosis and treatment of spontaneous pneumothorax. Arch Bronconeumol 2008;44:437–48 [in Spanish].

68. Chen W, Zhang C, Wang G, et al. The feasibility and safety of thoracoscopic surgery under epidural and/or local anesthesia for spontaneous pneumothorax: a meta-analysis. Wideochir Inne Tech Maloinwazyjne 2017;12:216–24.

69. Ahn HY, Kim YD, Cho JS, et al. Thoracoscopic surgery under epidural anesthesia for intractable secondary spontaneous pneumothorax. Asian J Surg 2017;40:285–9.

70. Tschopp JM, Brutsche M, Frey JG. Treatment of complicated spontaneous pneumothorax by simple talc pleurodesis under thoracoscopy and local anaesthesia. Thorax 1997;52(4):329–32.

Treatment of Pleural Effusions with Nonintubated Video-Assisted Thoracoscopic Surgery

Thamer Robert Qaqish, MD, Solange Cox, MD, Rebecca Carr, MBBS, Mark Katlic, MD*

KEYWORDS

• Pleural effusion • Minimally invasive thoracic surgery • Nonintubated thoracic surgery • VATS

KEY POINTS

• Nonintubated video-assisted thoracic surgery is a useful approach in the management of pleural effusions.
• Both simple and complex effusions are amenable to video-assisted thoracic surgery via a nonintubated approach.
• Techniques from conventional video-assisted thoracoscopic surgery are directly applicable in the nonintubated patient setting.

PLEURAL EFFUSIONS

The pleura is a serous membrane composed of pleural mesothelial cells arranged in 2 layers that line the surface of the lung (visceral pleura) and the internal surface of the thoracic cavity (parietal pleura).[1,2] These 2 layers of pleura are continuous with each other at the hilum, giving rise to the fluid-filled pleural cavity. Pleural fluid within this space promotes apposition of the lungs and the chest wall during respiration and lubricates opposing surfaces of the parietal and visceral pleura to facilitate rapid transmission of forces from the chest wall to the lungs during inspiration and expiration with minimal friction.[2,3]

Most pleural fluid is produced as an ultrafiltrate by the parietal pleura and the production of pleural fluid changes based on the hydrostatic, colloid, and tissue pressures within the pleural space and on the permeability of the pleural membrane.[2,4] The high capillary pressure associated with the systemic capillaries supplying the parietal pleura as compared with the intrapleural negative pressure produces a pressure gradient favoring filtration into the pleural space.[5–7] In contrast, low-pressure pulmonary circulation supplies the visceral pleura, producing a much less significant pressure gradient.[7,8] Pleural fluid is subsequently reabsorbed by the lymphatic stomata of the parietal pleura that open directly into the pleural space, which can increase the drainage flow rate by up to 20 times in response to increased production of pleural fluid.[1,2,4,9]

Under normal physiologic conditions, pleural fluid production is well balanced with the rate of absorption so as to maintain a low volume of fluid within this space, typically ranging between 0.1 and 0.2 mL/kg of pleural fluid per pleural cavity.[2,6] Maintaining pleural fluid volume within this range is critical to ensure appropriate respiratory function

Disclosure statement: The authors have nothing to disclose.
Department of Surgery, Sinai Hospital of Baltimore, 2435 West Belvedere Avenue, Suite 42, Baltimore, MD 21215, USA
* Corresponding author.
E-mail address: mkatlic@lifebridgehealth.org

and mechanical coupling of the lung and chest wall.[4,10,11] Disturbance in this careful fluid balance results in fluid accumulation within the pleural space ultimately causing pleural effusion development and respiratory dysfunction, as increases in pleural fluid decrease the amount of force transmitted between the thoracic wall and lung.[3] Pathologic accumulation of fluid within the pleural space may result from a pathologic decrease in the rate of pleural fluid reabsorption by the lymphatic system, a substantial increase in flow from the systemic vessels as a result of increased capillary endothelial permeability, and/or widening of the hydrostatic-oncotic pressure gradient favoring pleural fluid filtration into the pleural space.[5,6,9,10,12]

Pleural effusions are most often classified according to their protein composition as either transudative or exudative based on the criteria of Light and colleagues.[13,14] Transudative effusions are protein-poor effusions that most often result from alterations in Starling mechanisms that ultimately favor ultrafiltration of plasma and result in fluid overload, most commonly seen in congestive heart failure (increased hydrostatic pressure) and cirrhosis (decreased oncotic forces).[13] Conversely, exudative effusions are rich in protein that most often are the result of increased capillary permeability and/or impaired lymphatic drainage due to local proliferative (eg, malignancy) or inflammatory (eg, parapneumonic effusions) processes[15] (**Fig. 1**).

Clinically, this distinction is of vital importance, as most transudative effusions result from systemic diseases that cause alterations in cardiac, renal, or hepatic function, whereas exudative effusions indicate a local pathologic process and require further workup to definitely exclude an underlying malignancy. A malignant pleural effusion is defined by presence of neoplastic cells within the pleural space as a result of either a primary pleural malignancy or invasion of the pleura by metastatic neoplastic cells following hematogenous, lymphatic, or contiguous spread.[16–18] Most malignant pleural effusions are exudates and they most often develop as a result of tumor-induced lymphatic obstruction and/or tumor-induced increases in microvascular permeability.[3,10,19] Malignant pleural effusions are important clinically because they indicate a very poor prognosis, correlating with an overall survival of 3 to 12 months after diagnosis, and often lead to debilitating symptoms.[20]

MANAGEMENT OF PLEURAL EFFUSIONS
Thoracostomy Tube and Talc Slurry Instillation

Tube thoracostomy is a minimally invasive, low-cost bedside procedure. It is well tolerated in patients who are deemed inappropriate candidates for video-assisted thoracoscopic surgical (VATS) procedures. Talc slurry can be instilled through the tube, also as a bedside procedure to achieve pleurodesis.[21,22] Although this procedure is inexpensive and placement of the tube is simple, thoracostomy tubes do not allow for direct visualization of the pleural cavity. Because of lack of visualization, complete drainage may not be obtained. Furthermore, blind placement of talc for pleurodesis is not optimal and may lead to lower rates of pleurodesis compared with video-assisted procedures in which direct visualization is obtained.[23] In addition, the lack of visualization increases the chance that there may be a need for additional procedures for drainage. Patient satisfaction has been shown to be lower for bedside tube placement because the patient is awake and there is reported to be a higher amount of pain because this procedure is not done with intravenous sedation but only using local

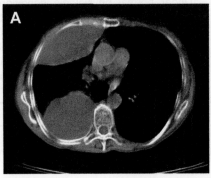 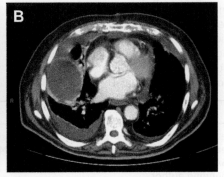

Fig. 1. (*A*) Multiloculated malignant pleural effusion due to ovarian cancer. (*B*) Multiloculated chronic hemothorax after cardiac surgery. (*From* Katlic MR. Five hundred seventy-six cases of video-assisted thoracic surgery using local anesthesia and sedation: lessons learned. J Am Coll Surg. 2018;226(1):59; with permission.)

anesthetic. A disadvantage of this procedure is that patients may likely go home with a chest tube in place that may have to remain in place for a longer period than those who have a VATS procedure.

Thoracentesis

This is a minimally invasive and cost-effective modality of treating pleural effusions. It is an outpatient procedure with low risk of complications.[24–26] Thoracentesis has a less important role in treating recurrent pleural effusions, as it does not prevent recurrence. There is no pleurodesis associated with this procedure, and because most of these effusions will recur, this method is not a definitive treatment method.[26] In addition, a tissue biopsy is usually not obtained with this procedure, making it a less desirable procedure than VATS, which can provide both diagnostic and therapeutic value.

Long-Term Indwelling Pleural Catheter

Placement of a long-term indwelling pleural PleurX catheter (CareFusion Corporation, San Diego, CA), is an overall well-tolerated procedure.[21,22,27] It is a minimally invasive, cost-effective, outpatient method for treatment of recurrent pleural effusions and involves more patient control over the drainage of their effusions.[21,27] The indwelling catheter is associated with a higher rate of complications, including catheter clogging, infections, and chronic pain at the catheter site.[26,27] These complications create the need for additional procedures. This method does not allow for obtaining any tissue for diagnosis nor does it facilitate the instillation of any form of chemical for pleurodesis.[26,27] **Table 1** outlines the advantages and disadvantages of various options to treat pleural effusions.

NONINTUBATED VIDEO-ASSISTED THORACOSCOPIC SURGERY

Our group has published a report previously on this topic and has outlined patient selection, preparation, and technique.[28–30]

Patient Selection and Preparation

In our prospectively maintained database, the cohort of patients we operated on have had large pleural effusions, pleural-based masses, early or midstage empyemas, or multiple lung nodules.[29] Advanced age is not a contraindication nor is weight, as our group has performed nonintubated VATS (NIVATS) on patients weighing in excess of 150 kg (**Fig. 2**). Furthermore, most patients are American Society of Anesthesiologists physical status classes 3 and 4. Extensive comorbidities are similarly not an absolute contraindication;

Table 1
Advantages and disadvantages of various options to treat pleural effusions

Treatment Method	Advantages	Disadvantages
Thoracoscopic chemical talc pleurodesis	Minimally invasive, can be outpatient Direct visualization, immediate and complete drainage High diagnostic yield of biopsy High pleurodesis rate Increased patient satisfaction	More costly than other methods Inpatient hospitalization May require tube thoracostomy following procedure
Tube thoracostomy and talc slurry	Minimally invasive Outpatient	Pain associated with indwelling tube May require inpatient hospitalization
Thoracentesis	Minimally invasive Outpatient	No pleurodesis achieved following procedure Frequent need for additional procedures
Long-term indwelling pleural catheter	Minimally invasive Outpatient	Chronic indwelling catheter Higher risk of infection Need for repeated drainage
Pleurectomy	High diagnostic yield of biopsy High pleurodesis rate	Invasive procedure Requires inpatient hospitalization

From Cox SE, Katlic MR. Non-intubated video-assisted thoracic surgery as the modality of choice for treatment of recurrent pleural effusions. Ann Transl Med 2015;3(8):103; with permission.

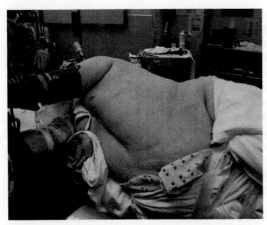

Fig. 2. Morbidly obese (172 kg) patient for whom we performed NIVATS drainage for an early multiloculated empyema.

however, this often requires consultation with the anesthesia provider preoperatively. Moreover, with the rotation of surgical technologists and circulating nurses, clear communication of anticipated steps and potential concerns between surgical team and operating room (OR) personnel also may facilitate a safe operation.

In general, the surgeon should have a solid foundation of the basics of minimally invasive surgery. In addition to good surgical technique and gentle handling of tissues, local anesthesia is of critical importance. Dose limitations should be respected and followed. Moreover, as with all thoracic surgery, careful personal preoperative review of all radiographic data is important for a successful operation.

TECHNIQUE

Sedation is achieved with combinations of midazolam, fentanyl, and propofol. Our anesthesia providers have full discretion of sedative administration but are aware of the depth of anesthesia required. Drainage of a pleural effusion with pleural biopsy via a single port may not require as deep sedation as a 2-port or 3-port lung biopsy. Oxygen is administered via nasal prongs and or face mask and full-face mask noninvasive ventilation also can be continued if necessary, to maintain oxygenation and ventilation. Hemodynamic, electrocardiographic, and end-tidal carbon dioxide capnography are continually assessed during the procedure. Flexible bronchoscopy is carried out if necessary, through the pharynx after direct lidocaine topical spray of the vocal cords. Full lateral positioning is necessary and is similar for other VATS procedures.

As a result of the obligatory pneumothorax, operative efficiency is encouraged and completing the procedure with a minimum of wasted steps is ideal for patient safety. The surgeon or resident should ensure that all suture material, thoracostomy tubes, and minimally invasive instruments are opened on the surgical technologist's table. There is surgeon preference regarding angled versus zero-degree laparoscope and suture material to secure the thoracostomy tubes; however, a minimum number of instruments are shown in **Fig. 3** that can be used for drainage procedures and lung biopsies.

Adequate local anesthesia for each layer of the chest wall cannot be overemphasized. Similarly, patience to allow time for the local anesthetic to work also should be accounted for. Comfortable and seamless port placement requires this especially when general anesthesia is not used. We repeatedly emphasize blunt spreading of tissues with alternating injections of anesthesia before through-and-through placement of the thoracic trocar. The senior author (MK) does not routinely use intercostal nerve blockade and carbon dioxide insufflation is also not practiced by our group.

As mentioned previously, clear and continual communication with the anesthesia provider and OR personnel will assist in an efficient and safe intubation as well as conversion to thoracotomy if required. Chest tube insertion via the thoracoscopic port site and occlusive dressings on other sites are required before placing the patient supine for intubation. An alternative is placement of a laryngeal mask airway while the patient is still

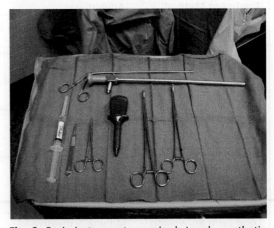

Fig. 3. Basic instruments required. Local anesthetic, scalpel blade, Crile clamp, thoracoscopic port to permit a 10-mm laparoscope, and up cup biopsy forceps (23–33 cm). Laparoscopic staplers (not shown) and laparoscopic scissors (not shown) also may be used for lung biopsy and pericardial drainage, respectively.

lateral. Thus far, the senior author has not had any thoracotomy conversions or intraoperative intubations.

Elective patients may be discharged the same day from the post-anesthesia care unit or go home the following day. Those who go home the same day, do so with a Mini-Atrium Dry Seal Chest Drain (Atrium Medical, Hudson, NH). Tube thoracostomy removal is performed in the outpatient clinic when appropriate.

TECHNICAL CONSIDERATIONS

Depending on the intrathoracic pathology being examined, 1, 2, or 3 port sites may be used.

Pleural drainage procedures and pleural biopsies can be performed with a single port. Biopsy instruments can be passed alongside the thoracoscopic trocar through the same incision (**Fig. 4**). If an early, multiloculated empyema is encountered, a second port site can be fashioned for pneumolysis using an instrument or finger. Posteriorly, the intercostal spaces are narrowest. One end of the army-navy retractor may be passed through the incision parallel to the ribs and twisted perpendicularly to wedge the posterior interspace open and expand the area. It will not immediately return to its original shape. This may offer added room for instrument use between ribs posteriorly. Last, talc insufflation and insertion of a PleurX catheter (CareFusion Corporation) may be performed at the end of the case using the single incision.

Pericardial drainage and biopsy can be performed using a 2-port or 3-port approach. If the patient is hemodynamically stable and/or there is a concomitant intrathoracic pathology that

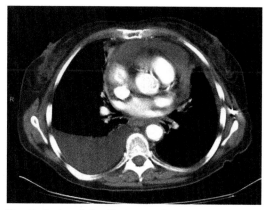

Fig. 5. Pericardial effusion with coexisting pleural effusion.

requires evaluation, pericardial drainage and biopsy can be safely performed under sedation (**Fig. 5**). The laparoscope may be placed posteriorly inferior to the scapula and a second port immediately anterior to the pericardium. A third port may be placed superiorly between the 2 existing ports if the lung needs to be retracted or compressed to safely expose the pericardium and phrenic nerve. A long-handled 15-blade can be inserted under direct vision anterior to the pericardium. A grasper can be placed alongside the camera port, while endoscopic or long-handled Metzenbaum scissors can be used from the anterior port to remove the pericardial biopsy.

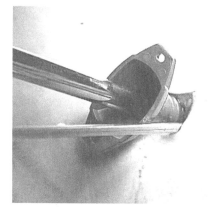

Fig. 4. Technique used to maximize instrument use through a single incision. The surgeon may also slide the thoracoscopic port out of the body toward the camera head, along the camera shaft and this may allow the adjacent instrument better and more precise movement.

Table 2	
List of procedures performed in patients receiving nonintubated video-assisted thorascopic surgery	
Procedure	**n**
Drain effusion/pleural biopsy (n = 368)	
With talc insufflation	302
Without talc insufflation	66
Drain empyema	112
Lung biopsy	56
Evacuate chronic hemothorax	23
Pericardial window	10
Treat chylothorax	2
Drain lung abscess	2
Treat pneumothorax	2
Biopsy mediastinal mass	1

From Katlic MR. Five hundred seventy-six cases of video-assisted thoracic surgery using local anesthesia and sedation: lessons learned. J Am Coll Surg. 2018;226(1):62; with permission.

Table 3
Comparison of outcomes with various treatment regimens for recurrent pleural effusions

Treatment Method	Average Cost	Symptom Relief	Need for Further Procedures	Pleurodesis Rate	Mortality	Morbidity[a]	Diagnostic Yield of Biopsy	Length of Hospital Stay, d
Thoracoscopic talc pleurodesis[b]	$780	+++	<10%	>90%	<0.5%	2+	+++	0–1
Thoracoscopic talc pleurodesis[c]	$780	+++	<10%	>90%	<0.5%	2+	+++	6 ± 4
Tube thoracostomy and talc slurry	$355	+++	16%	55%–90%	0%	1+	–	6
Thoracentesis	$84	++	98%	2%	0%	<1	+	–
Indwelling pleural catheter	$250	+++	23%	42%–58%	0%	1+	–	1–3±2
Pleurectomy	$3500	+++	<1%	99%	10%–19%	5+	+++	8–9

Abbreviations: ++, indicates intermediate level of success; +++, indicates high level of success.
[a] Indicates morbidity as evaluated on a scale of 1 to 5.
[b] Indicates video-assisted thoracoscopic surgery using local anesthetic and intravenous sedation.
[c] Indicates video-assisted thoracoscopic surgery with intubation.
From Cox SE, Katlic MR. Non-intubated video-assisted thoracic surgery as the modality of choice for treatment of recurrent pleural effusions. Ann Transl Med 2015;3(8):103; with permission.

Lung biopsies may be performed under sedation in a manner similar to single lung ventilation; however, lung compression is important to improve visualization of the lung biopsy target. For example, the elbow of the reticulated stapler can be used to compress lung tissue while negotiating the distal tips underneath grasped lung tissue. Bulky endocatch bags are difficult to negotiate within a smaller intrathoracic space and are not used. Solitary lung nodules not immediately peripheral are difficult to find.

The senior author has published a large series of NIVATS in which 529 patients underwent 576 operations[29] for a variety of diagnoses that included both benign (n = 139) and malignant (n = 224) pleural effusions, empyema (n = 112), lung disease (n = 56), and chronic hemothorax (n = 23). Most of the procedures involved drainage with pleural biopsies (n = 368, 302 with talc pleurodesis). Patient age ranged from 21 to 104 years, and patient weight from 40 to 181 kg. Mean operative time was 26 minutes (8–111 minutes range). No patient required intraoperative intubation or conversion to thoracotomy. One lung biopsy was aborted because of hypercarbia and agitation but was eventually successfully completed 2 days later using general anesthesia and single lung ventilations. From 112 patients who underwent NIVATS for empyema, 3 required a subsequent procedure for empyema. Fifty patients were discharged on the same day of the procedure (42 with pleural effusions and 8 with chronic hemothoraces). A list of procedures is provided in **Table 2**.

Although not as commonly performed, lobectomies and nonanatomical lung resections are increasingly being performed using NIVATS. In a retrospective series reported by Al Ghamdi and colleagues,[31] 31 VATS lobectomies performed via general anesthesia were compared with 31 lobectomies performed in nonintubated patients. Short-term perioperative outcomes, such as operative stay and duration of tube thoracostomy drainage, were similar; however, mean lymph node yield was greater for intubated patients (18.0 vs 12.6).

Moreover, Liu and colleagues[32] reported comparable and even improved short-term perioperative outcomes, such as hospital stay and overall drainage volume, in patients who underwent nonintubated anatomic VATS resections (lobectomy n = 119) under local anesthesia versus general endotracheal anesthesia (lobectomy n = 163). Furthermore, in this review, lymph node yield was similar in both groups. Patients with a history of thoracic surgery, severe coronary artery disease, unstable asthma, history of tuberculosis or other diseases that causes pleural adhesions and those who were converted from nonintubated to intubated (n = 9) were excluded from each group for comparison. **Table 3** outlines a comparison of outcomes with various treatment regimens for recurrent pleural effusions.

Patients tolerate NIVATS well with minimal pain and recall. Respiratory effort postoperatively is relatively strong and the patients tolerate the obligatory pneumothorax as long as an hour in the senior author's experience. NIVATS using local anesthesia and sedation is well tolerated, safe, and valuable for a number of indications.

REFERENCES

1. Finley DJ, Rusch VW. Anatomy of the pleura. Thorac Surg Clin 2011;21:157–63, vii.
2. Wang NS. Anatomy of the pleura. Clin Chest Med 1998;19:229–40.
3. Zocchi L. Physiology and pathophysiology of pleural fluid turnover. Eur Respir J 2002;20:1545–58.
4. Negrini D, Moriondo A. Pleural function and lymphatics. Acta Physiol (Oxf) 2013;207:244–59.
5. Mehran JR, Deslauriers J. Anatomy and physiology of the pleural space. In: Patterson GA, Cooper JD, Deslauries J, et al, editors. Pearson's thoracic and esophageal surgery. Philadelphia: Churchill Livingstone-Elsevier; 2008. p. 1001–7.
6. Yalcin NG, Choong CK, Eizenberg N. Anatomy and pathophysiology of the pleura and pleural space. Thorac Surg Clin 2013;23:1–10.
7. Lai-Fook SJ. Pleural mechanics and fluid exchange. Physiol Rev 2004;84:385–410.
8. Deatrick KB, Long J, Chang AC. Thoracic wall, pleura, mediastinum, and lung. In: Doherty GM, editor. Current surgical diagnosis and treatment. New York: McGraw-Hill; 2015. p. 331–89.
9. Feller-Kopman D, Light R. Pleural disease. N Engl J Med 2018;378:740–51.
10. Sahn SA. The pathophysiology of pleural effusions. Annu Rev Med 1990;41:7–13.
11. Froudarakis ME. Diagnostic work-up of pleural effusions. Respiration 2008;75:4–13.
12. Bhatnagar R, Maskell N. The modern diagnosis and management of pleural effusions. BMJ 2015;351: h4520.
13. Porcel JM, Light RW. Pleural effusions. Dis Mon 2013;59:29–57.
14. Light RW. Pleural effusions. Med Clin North Am 2011;95:1055–70.
15. Na MJ. Diagnostic tools of pleural effusion. Tuberc Respir Dis (Seoul) 2014;76:199–210.
16. Heffner JE, Klein JS. Recent advances in the diagnosis and management of malignant pleural effusions. Mayo Clin Proc 2008;83:235–50.

17. Heffner JE. Diagnosis and management of malignant pleural effusions. Respirology 2008;13:5–20.

18. Jantz MA, Antony VB. Pathophysiology of the pleura. Respiration 2008;75:121–33.

19. Sahn SA. Malignancy metastatic to the pleura. Clin Chest Med 1998;19:351–61.

20. Kastelik JA. Management of malignant pleural effusion. Lung 2013;191:165–75.

21. Rusch VW, Mountain C. Thoracoscopy under regional anesthesia for the diagnosis and management of pleural disease. Am J Surg 1987;154:274–8.

22. Pompeo E. Awake thoracic surgery—is it worth the trouble? Semin Thorac Cardiovasc Surg 2012;24: 106–14.

23. Rahman NM, Ali NJ, Brown G, et al. Local anaesthetic thoracoscopy: British Thoracic Society Pleural Disease Guideline 2010. Thorax 2010;65(Suppl 2): ii54–60.

24. Migliore M, Giuliano R, Aziz T, et al. Four-step local anesthesia and sedation for thoracoscopic diagnosis and management of pleural diseases. Chest 2002;121:2032–5.

25. Danby CA, Adebonojo SA, Moritz DM. Video-assisted talc pleurodesis for malignant pleural effusions utilizing local anesthesia and I.V. sedation. Chest 1998;113:739–42.

26. Harris RJ, Kavuru MS, Rice TW, et al. The diagnostic and therapeutic utility of thoracoscopy: a review. Chest 1995;108:828–41.

27. Olden AM, Holloway R. Treatment of malignant pleural effusion: PleurX catheter or talc pleurodesis? A cost-effectiveness analysis. J Palliat Med 2010;13:59–65.

28. Cox SE, Katlic MR. Non-intubated video-assisted thoracic surgery as the modality of choice for treatment of recurrent pleural effusions. Ann Transl Med 2015;3:25–9.

29. Katlic MR. Five hundred seventy-six cases of video-assisted thoracic surgery using local anesthesia and sedation: lessons learned. J Am Coll Surg 2018;226: 58–63.

30. Katlic MR. Video-assisted thoracic surgery utilizing local anesthesia and sedation: how I teach it. Ann Thorac Surg 2017;104:727–30.

31. Al Ghamdi ZM, Lynhiavu L, Moon YK, et al. Comparison of non-intubated versus intubated video-assisted thoracoscopic lobectomy for lung cancer. J Thorac Dis 2018;10:4236–43.

32. Liu J, Cui F, Pompeo E, et al. The impact of non-intubated versus intubated anaesthesia on early outcomes of video-assisted thoracoscopic anatomical resection in non-small-cell lung cancer: a propensity score matching analysis. Eur J Cardiothorac Surg 2016;50:920–5.

Nonintubated Uniportal Video-Assisted Thoracic Surgery for Chest Infections

Marcello Migliore, MD, PhD, FETCS

KEYWORDS

- Chest infection • Empyema • VATS • Minimally invasive thoracic surgery
- Uniportal thoracic surgery • Non intubated • Awake surgery

KEY POINTS

- Video-assisted thoracic surgery (VATS) is accepted as a useful treatment option for stages II to III pleural empyema.
- Uniportal VATS has all the potential to become the standard of care for stages II to III pleural empyema.
- Nonintubated VATS is indicated in very ill patients.
- Nonintubated anesthesia is easier to perform using uniportal VATS.

INTRODUCTION

Chest infection is a health care problem in many regions of the world; in particular, lower respiratory tract infection is the fourth most common cause of death globally and one of the major causes of postoperative death.[1–3] Chest infection affects principally the lung, and the main causes include virus and bacteria.

Chest infections can affect people of all ages, including children, the elderly, and smokers. Moreover, people who are already ill (with chronic obstructive pulmonary disease or heart, liver, or renal disease) and older people are most likely of developing a chest infection.

Clinically, patients develop high temperature (fever) above 38C°; chest pain, which is made worse when breathing; dry cough; chills; excessive sweating, particularly at night; shortness of breath; and general sense of feeling unwell.

Because 10% of patients with pleural effusion due to pneumonia develop loculation or progress to empyema,[3] thoracic surgeons often are involved when more life-threatening complications appear, such as empyema and lung abscesses.

EMPYEMA

The incidence of pleural empyema has increased since 1990, and it has affected more than 65,000 patients each year in the United States and United Kingdom.[4] From 1996 to 2008, the hospitalization for pleural empyema increased from 3.0 to 5.9 per 100,000 in the United States population. Postpneumonic pleural empyema, the most common form of pleural empyema (60%), is increasing in North America and Europe and is recognized as a major cause of morbidity and prolonged hospital stay. The second most common cause of pleural empyema is postsurgical (30%), for example, pleural empyema caused by postoperative bronchopleural fistula or in pneumonotomies patients. Despite medical treatment, patients suffering with pleural empyema develop significant morbidity and mortality. The American Thoracic

Disclosure Statement: The author has nothing to disclose.
Section of Thoracic Surgery, Department of Surgery and Medical Specialities, University of Catania, Policlinic University Hospital, Catania, Italy
E-mail address: mmiglior@unict.it

Society divides pleural empyema in 3 stages, as in listed **Table 1**.

Diagnosis usually is performed during the first stage and it is based on the results of a thoracocentesis, which shows a purulent fluid, glucose less than 50 mg/dL, high protein greater than 30 mg/dL, pH less than 7.2, and lactate dehydrogenase greater than 1000 IU/L. Treatment is generally nonsurgical.[5,6]

The fibrinopurulent stage (stage II) has been characterized by a thick fluid and thick fibrin strands (**Fig. 1**), pH less than7.2, lactate dehydrogenase greater than 1000 IU/L, glucose less than 60 mg/dL, positive culture or presence of suppuration, and increased loculations in the pleural cavity. Fibrinopurulent empyema changes into an organizing stage within 7 days to 10 days of symptom initiation. In addition, lung entrapment should be suspected when the pleural infection process is known to have been ongoing for longer than 10 days to 14 days. The 3 stages of pleural empyema require an individualized treatment, but only the second and third stages are definitely for thoracic surgeons.

LUNG ABSCESS

A lung abscess is a rare complication of pneumonia and is mostly seen in people who have a serious, preexisting illness or those with a history of severe alcohol misuse. The symptoms of a lung abscess are the same as those of severe pneumonia. In addition, the patients could start to cough up unpleasant-smelling phlegm and experience swelling in fingers and toes. Most cases of lung abscesses can be treated using antibiotics. This usually involves an initial course of intravenous (IV) antibiotics (directly into a vein through a drip) followed by oral antibiotics (tablets) for 4 weeks to 6 weeks. Most people who have a lung abscess experience an improvement in their symptoms within 3 days to 4 days. It is important to finish a recommended course of antibiotics, even if feeling perfectly healthy, to prevent reinfection of the lungs. Approximately 10% of people require invasive treatment because they fail to respond to the antibiotics. Surgery is rare because

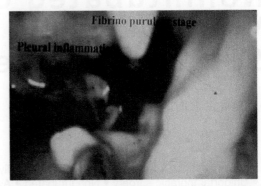

Fig. 1. Uniportal VATS. Intraoperative photo, stage II empyema. Pus, fibrin, and pleural inflammation are visible.

many patients with lung abscesses are now being drained under guidance of computed tomography (CT) scan without the necessity of removing the affected section of the lung.

AIM OF THE ARTICLE

In the past decennium, the broadened use of uniportal video-assisted thoracic surgery (VATS) and nonintubated surgery has changed considerably surgical treatment of pleural empyema. Nonintubated VATS has been reported safe and feasible in many circumstances, such as major lung resection, pneumothorax, wedge resection, and lung volume reduction surgery.[7]

This article has been written with the intention to answer the following 2 questions:

1. Is nonintubated surgery appropriate for VATS treatment of pleural empyema?
2. What is the best VATS approach for nonintubated surgery in the treatment of pleural empyema?

NONINTUBATED ANESTHESIA FOR PLEURAL EMPYEMA

Until the advent of VATS, curative surgery for pleural empyema was mainly performed under general anesthesia with a double-lumen tube. It is evident that anesthetic management for awake surgery in patients with pleural empyema is more challenging than under general anesthesia, requiring experience and careful patient selection. Nonintubated VATS certainly represents a step forward, and it is to be considered suitable for selected patients, with many advantages. In general, the absence of general anesthesia results in early postoperative pulmonary reexpansion, faster recovery, and a decrease in hospitalization.[7–10] Several techniques have

Table 1	
The 3 stages of empyema	
American Thoracic Society Stage	**Type of Empyema**
First stage	Acute–exudative
Second stage	Fibrinopurulent
Third stage	Organizing–cortical

been described to perform an operation without an endotracheal tube in patients with pleural empyema. Buckingham and colleagues[11] described in 1950 experience with of 617 thoracic surgery procedures performed under thoracic epidural anesthesia, and in 1954 Vischnevski[12] reported a series 600 thoracic surgery procedures performed under local anesthesia. Paravertebral block has also been reported to perform nonintubated VATS.

During awake surgery, the iatrogenic pneumothorax allows a sufficient lung collapse, allowing it to work smoothly. Moreover, the presence of spontaneous breathing and mobility of the diaphragm counteract the possibility of a mediastinal shift.[8] The main advantage of nonintubated surgery for empyema is the particular importance in unstable patients with multiple comorbidities or in patients allergic to general anesthesia. Rare reports have demonstrated that VATS decortication could effectively manage empyema in awake patients using epidural or paravertebral nerve block. It was even suggested that spontaneous lung ventilation resulted in easier dissection during the operation, resulting in lower postoperative morbidity.[13]

Patients must be informed of their rights & responsibilities before consenting, and accurate perioperative care is of paramount importance for successful patient management.

After positioning, the patient is continuously monitored for the duration of the surgery, with pulse oximeter, electrocardiogram, invasive blood pressure, bispectral index, and arterial blood gases. Midazolam, 1.5 mg, and fentanyl, 50 μg, also are administered. The objective is to keep the bispectral (BIS) index between 75 and 85. Patients are kept at spontaneous breathing with oxygen saturation as measured by pulse oximetry 95% to 96% (nasal cannula fraction of inspired oxygen 30%). Arterial blood gases are monitored intraoperatively and Acetaminophen (paracetamol), 1 g, is administered as an analgesic. Acetaminophen (paracetamol), 1 g, is administered as an analgesic.

Although several anesthetic techniques have been reported for VATS in pleural empyema, in 1998, the author introduced a 4-step local anesthesia and sedation for thoracic procedures with excellent results in many patients.[14–18] During surgery the anesthetist continuously monitored noninvasive blood pressure, electrocardiogram, and oxygen saturation. Facial mask was used to administer oxygen, and IV cannula inserted. Premedication was performed with droperidol and atropine before operation. Sedation was maintained by diazepam given a few minutes before local anesthesia, using ropicavaine in 4 different steps.

The first step was the injection of local anesthetic made at the site of the 2 cm above and parallel to the rib and the dissection started though the subcutaneous tissue.

The second step was the injection of local anesthetic at the aponeurosis of the thoracic muscles.

After the muscle is opened, the third step consisted of palpating the rib and make the incision down to the rib.

The fourth and final step consisted of anesthetizing the pleura by infiltration through the intercostal muscles for 3 cm to 4 cm. The incision was then made on the superior border of the rib. Just before the pleural is opened, another IV bolus of propofol was administered (30–60 mg IV in 10–15 s).

Decreased oxygen desaturation was treated with increasing oxygen flow. When necessary, propofol was injected by demand and plasma expanders were used to treat hypotension secondary to propofol. The instrumentation and the drug for general anesthesia were always available in the operating room.

OPERATIVE TECHNIQUE

It is mandatory before surgery to have the correct empyema stage assessment, which must be done with a clear description of the radiographic aspect and with a CT scan, which can help to locate the presence of a thick pleura, which is a pathognomonic sign of stage 3 empyema, as shown in **Fig. 2**.

The surgical team is formed by the primary surgeon, a first assistant (not always necessary), and a scrub nurse. Although in the early days, the

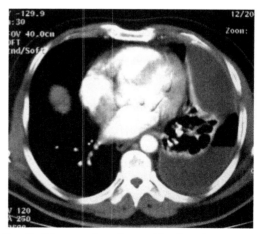

Fig. 2. CT scan of patient with pleural empyema stages II to III. A thick visceral pleura is visible (*whitish border*).

classic thoracoscope was used to make diagnosis and treat early fibrinopurulent stage, in 1998, the author stopped the use of the classic thoracoscope and started using VATS performed through a port or flexible trocar to perform many thoracic procedures, including empyema.[14–17] The preferred position is posterolateral but, depending on the specific location of the lesion and general condition, the supine or anterolateral position could be used.

Although today a minithoracotomy of 4-cm to 6-cm incision is called uniportal in many centers, the author uses a 2-cm incision to insert a flexible port of 20 mm. Opening of the pleura may not be straightforward because it is often thick. After the pleura is entered, the index finger is used to lyse the possible adhesions of the lung to the chest wall. Intrathoracic treatment is different according to the findings of stage II empyema: debridement and stage III empyema: lung decortication.

The specimen is always sent for microbiological and pathologic examinations because cancer and mesothelioma could be hidden by an empyema. A chest drain (sometimes 2 drains) is inserted through the incision under visual control and connected to an underwater-seal bottle system. The author has developed a double chest drain for uniportal VATS. After surgery, the patient is observed at the recovery room for 3 hours. A chest radiograph is taken in the recovery room and the patient is transferred in the surgical ward. Postoperatively, chest radiographs are taken daily to ensure full lung expansion and to check for any pneumothorax or residual effusion. The chest drainage is under suction for at least 48 hours. Although in the author's unit, fast-track rules have been recently followed for many operations, in cases of pleural effusion, the tube was removed when the drainage was less than 150 mL daily.

The author performed surgery for stages II to III pleural empyema under awake surgery in 54 patients; of those, thoracic débridement for stage II empyema was performed in 42 patients and lung decortication for stage III empyema in 12 patients. One patient has been converted to open minithoracotomy for bleeding and was intubated with a single-lumen tube. There was neither mortality nor major morbidity. Hospitalization averaged 6 days. One patient had recurrence of the empyema at subsequent follow-ups.[19,20]

DISCUSSION AND ANSWER TO THE TWO QUESTIONS

VATS has become a common and globally accepted surgical approach for a variety of thoracic diseases. Conventionally, it is performed under tracheal intubation with double-lumen tube or bronchial blocker to achieve single-lung ventilation. Generally, it is performed with 2-port or 4-port accesses.[21–24]

VATS has been demonstrated to be superior to open decortication (or chest tube drainage) for the management of adults with primary empyema in terms of postoperative morbidity, complications, and length of hospital stay and has equivalent resolution compared with open decortication. Additionally, VATS resulted in reduced postoperative pain ($P<.0001$) and complications, including atelectasis ($P = .006$), prolonged air-leak ($P = .0003$), sepsis ($P = .03$), and 30-day mortality ($P = .02$). Another study performed in 106 patients demonstrated that patients treated with VATS débridement or decortication spent less time in the hospital, and the conversion rate to open procedure for stage III empyema was only 19%, which encourages considering VATS débridement/decortication as a first-choice treatment.[25]

The guidelines produce by the British Thoracic Society suggest surgical treatment in patients with nonresolved pleural empyema with a maximum period of 7 days without resolution.[26] Early referral to surgery is a key factor for a successful operation of pleural empyema by VATS approach. Conversion from VATS to thoracotomy range from 5.6% to 61% but increases from 22% to 86% between day 12 and day 16 of presentation, and patients with a symptom duration of less than 4 weeks had better early results compared with a symptom duration of more than 4 weeks.[27,28] Stefani and colleagues[29] demonstrated that the probability of thoracotomy increased from 28% to 81% if the operation was performed within 10 days or after a delay of 30 days to 40 days. International guidelines recognize, however, a definite role for VAT in stage III pleural empyema.

The guidelines proposed by the European Association for Cardio-Thoracic Surgery preferred VATS in patients with stages II to III pleural empyema with the omission of stage III empyema with more than 5 weeks symptomatic clinical history.[30] VATS decortication has also been reported to successfully manage tuberculous empyema. Irrespective of the pleural empyema stage, some patients have a hidden chest malignancy[17]; therefore, some investigators suggest performing bronchoscopy in all patients with pleural empyema to rule out possible cancers that could influence the approach. Although the advancement in imaging techniques and therapeutic tools, it is evident that guidelines to use nonintubated VATS for pleural empyema do not exist. Nevertheless, experience teaches that in the treatment of chest infection, there are circumstances where it is preferred to perform nonintubated VATS: (1) critically ill patients and (2) stage 2 empyema. Although it is not possible to suggest objective criteria to define the point at which a patient should proceed to nonintubated surgery, patients with purulent fluid and/or loculations at presentation or with residual sepsis syndrome and persistent pleural collection despite drainage and antibiotics are considered more likely to benefit from surgical debridement of the pleural cavity. The most frequent complications are prolonged air leak, bleeding, recurrence or persistence of the disease, surgical wound infection, and residual pleural space. The 30-day postoperative mortality ranges from 1.3% to 6.6%.

IS NONINTUBATED ANESTHESIA APPROPRIATE FOR VIDEO-ASSISTED THORACIC SURGERY TREATMENT OF PLEURAL EMPYEMA?

There is no dogma that ascertain the no-usefulness of nonintubated anesthesia for VATS treatment of pleural empyema; nevertheless, the decision is often based on surgeon experience with awake surgery and the patient's clinical status, such as fever, leukocytosis, chest radiography, and chest CT.

It is known that nonintubated thoracic surgery offers many advantages to the patient.[31,32] Awake surgery is of particular importance in unstable patients with multiple comorbidities or in patients allergic to general anesthesia. Moreover, patients have a significantly reduced incidence of postoperative respiratory complications, including pneumonia and acute respiratory distress syndrome. Awake thoracic surgery also may reduce stress hormone response, attenuate the impact on the immune system, and lower the impact on postoperative lymphocyte response.[33]

Although for some physicians it could sound unethical, nowadays nonintubated anesthesia should be also the preferred choice in patients with a high risk for ventilator dependency. In addition, intubation-related airway trauma to teeth or vocal cords can also occur during intubation. Awake thoracic surgery also resulted in faster postoperative recovery and lower complication rates, and patients can display effective cough minutes after surgery. Patients have no intubation-associated discomfort, such as a sore throat and can return more quickly to daily activities, including drinking, eating, and walking.[10]

From the surgical point of view, it was been suggested that spontaneous lung ventilation resulted in easier dissection and less postoperative morbidity. In a recent experience of 33 patients with stage II pleural empyema and coronary artery disease and reduced left ventricular ejection fraction, 12 were treated using single-port nonintubated video-assisted flexible thoracoscopy surgery. The author found that chest tube drainage days, postoperative fever subsided days, postoperative hospital days, and total length of stay were significantly shorter in the single-port nonintubated video-assisted flexible thoracoscopy surgery decortications group (P value = .0027, .0001, .0009, and .0065, respectively). Morbidities were low, and mortality was significantly low (P value = .0319) in single-port nonintubated video-assisted flexible thoracoscopy surgery decortications.[34]

Furthermore, although the developing concept of nonintubated surgery imposes the need to clarify its possible indication in pleural empyema, nowadays it is important to answer a second question:

WHAT IS THE BEST VATS APPROACH FOR NONINTUBATED VATS IN THE TREATMENT OF PLEURAL EMPYEMA?

What seems to be evident is that the introduction of uniportal VATS certainly facilitated the use of awake nonintubated surgery in pleural empyema, because the main advantage of uniportal VATS is that it is necessary to use local anesthesia only in the small portion of the chest where the incision is made.[16,35–42]

There is no rule for the decision about the type of VATS approach; it is based mainly on surgeon experience, subjective opinion, and available equipment. Because since 1998 the author has performed uniportal VATS approach for pleural empyema, the author's personal experience suggests that surgery should be performed by experienced surgeons for many reasons—first, because the empyema sac often extends deep in the mediastinum in close contact with important structures like the esophagus, superior vena cava, and aorta, and second, because the surgeon must have the experience to decide when to convert to open thoracotomy for a formal decortication. Often a formal posterolateral thoracotomy is not necessary but most of the time a video-assisted minithoracotomy of 10 cm is sufficient to treat many intraoperative complications. Some surgeons speculated that spontaneous ventilation surgery, maintaining the lung expanded, facilitated identification of the correct plane and dissection, thus resulting in lesser surgical injury and postoperative air leaks.[43,44]

In the modern era, surgery for pleural empyema could be performed under awake surgery, preferably using uniportal VATS in opposition to the principle of old-style thoracic surgery, which required a double-lumen tube. Although the advantages seem evident, it is still early to conclude the benefits of this technique, because often there is the need for randomized controlled trials.

The future directions of nonintubated VATS for pleural empyema should focus on its long-term outcomes. Moreover, it is probably necessary to start a worldwide educating and training program for thoracic surgeons and anesthesiologists to allow an increase in awake surgical options in caring for patients with stages II to III empyema.

REFERENCES

1. Ahmed RA, Marrie TJ, Huang JQ. Thoracic empyema in patients with community-acquired pneumonia. Am J Med 2006;119:877–83.
2. Troeger C, Blacker B, Khalil IA. Estimates of the global, regional, and national morbidity, mortality, and aetiologies of lower respiratory infections in 195 countries, 1990–2016: a systematic analysis for the Global Burden of Disease Study 2016. Lancet Infect Dis 2018;18:1191–210.
3. Subotic D, Lardinois D, Hojski A. Minimally invasive thoracic surgery for empyema. Breathe (Sheff) 2018; 14:302–10.
4. Toker A, Hazer S, Rathinam S. Surgery for pleural sepsis. In: Modi P, editor. Perspectives in cardiothoracic surgery, vol. 1. London: Society for Cardiothoracic Surgery in Great Britain and Ireland; 2016. p. 122–9.
5. Light RW. Management of parapneumonic effusions. Arch Intern Med 1981;141:1339–41.
6. Cameron R, Davies HR. Intra-pleural fibrinolytic therapy versus conservative management in the treatment of adult parapneumonic effusions and empyema. Cochrane Database Syst Rev 2008;(2): CD002312.
7. Mineo TC, Migliore M. Innovation in awake VATS. Video Assist Thorac Surg 2018;3(2). https://doi.org/10.21037/vats.2018.01.05.
8. Mineo TC, Ambrogi V. A glance at the history of uniportal video-assisted thoracic surgery. J Vis Surg 2017;3:157.
9. Mineo TC, Tacconi F. From "awake" to "monitored anesthesia care" thoracic surgery: a 15 year evolution. Thorac Cancer 2014;5:1–13.
10. Gabor K, Castillo M. Nonintubated anesthesia in thoracic surgery: general issues. Ann Transl Med 2015;3:110.
11. Buckingham WW, Beatty AJ, Brasher CA, et al. The technique of administering epidural anesthesia in thoracic surgery. Dis Chest 1950;17:561–8.
12. Vischnevski AA. Local anesthesia in thoracic surgery: lungs, heart and esophagus. Minerva Anestesiol 1954;20:432–5.
13. Tacconi F, Pompeo E, Fabbi E, et al. Awake video-assisted pleural decortication for empyema thoracis. Eur J Cardiothorac Surg 2010;37: 594–601.
14. Migliore M, Deodato G. A single-trocar technique for minimally-invasive surgery of the chest. Surg Endosc 2001;15:899–901.
15. Migliore M, Giuliano R, Deodato G. Video assisted thoracic surgery through a single port. Thoracic surgery and Interdisciplinary Symposium on the threshold of the third Millennium. An international continuing medical education Programme. Naples, Italy, May 11-13, 2000. p. 29–30. Available at: http://xoomer.virgilio.it/naples2000/index1.html.
16. Migliore M, Giuliano R, Aziz T, et al. Four-step local anesthesia and sedation for thoracoscopic diagnosis and management of pleural diseases. Chest 2002;121:2032–5.
17. Migliore M. Efficacy and safety of single-trocar technique for minimally invasive surgery of the chest in the treatment of noncomplex pleural disease. J Thorac Cardiovasc Surg 2003;126: 1618–23.
18. Migliore M, Calvo D, Criscione A, et al. Uniportal video assisted thoracic surgery: summary of experience, mini-review and perspectives. J Thorac Dis 2015;7(9):E378.
19. Migliore M, Deodato G. Thoracoscopic surgery, video-thoracoscopic surgery, or VATS: a confusion in definition. Ann Thorac Surg 2000;69:1990–1.
20. Migliore M. Initial history of uniportal VATS. Ann Thorac Surg 2016;101:412–3.
21. Zahid I, Nagendran M, Routledge T, et al. Comparison of video-assisted thoracoscopic surgery and open surgery in the management of primary empyema. Curr Opin Pulm Med 2011;17:255–9.
22. Drain AJ, Ferguson JI, Sayeed R, et al. Definitive management of advanced empyema by two-window video-assisted surgery. Asian Cardiovasc Thorac Ann 2007;15:238–9.
23. Waller DA, Rengarajan A. Thoracoscopic decortication: a role for video-assisted surgery in chronic postpneumonic pleural empyema. Ann Thorac Surg 2001;71:1813–6.
24. Wilson H, Mohite P, Hall A, et al. Timing and efficacy of VATS debridement in the treatment of parapneumonic empyema. Arch Pulmonol Respir Care 2016; 2(1):16–9.
25. Chambers A, Routledge T, Dunning J, et al. Is video-assisted thoracoscopic surgical decortication superior to open surgery in the management of adults with primary empyema? Interact Cardiovasc Thorac Surg 2010;11:171–7.

26. Davies CW, Gleeson FV, Davies RJ. BTS guidelines for the management of pleural infection. Thorax 2003;58(Suppl. 2):ii18–28.

27. Lardinois D, Gock M, Pezzetta E, et al. Delayed referral and Gram-negative organisms increase the conversion thoracotomy rate in patients undergoing video-assisted thoracoscopic surgery for empyema. Ann Thorac Surg 2005;79:1851–6.

28. Chung JH, Lee SH, Kim KT, et al. Optimal timing of thoracoscopic drainage and decortication for empyema. Ann Thorac Surg 2014;97:224–9.

29. Stefani A, Aramini B, della Casa G, et al. Preoperative predictors of successful surgical treatment in the management of parapneumonic empyema. Ann Thorac Surg 2013;96:1812–9.

30. Scarci M, Abah U, Solli P, et al. EACTS expert consensus statement for surgical management of pleural empyema. Eur J Cardiothorac Surg 2015; 48:642.

31. Liu YJ, Hung MH, Hsu HH, et al. Effects on respiration of nonintubated anesthesia in thoracoscopic surgery under spontaneous ventilation. Ann Transl Med 2015;3:107.

32. Gelzinis TA, Sullivan EA. Non-intubated general anesthesia for video-assisted thoracoscopic surgery. J Cardiothorac Vasc Anesth 2017;31:407–8.

33. Mineo TC, Sellitri F, Vanni G, et al. Immunological and inflammatory impact of non-intubated lung metastasectomy. Int J Mol Sci 2017;18:1466.

34. Hsiao CH, Chen CC, Chen SS. Modified single-port non-intubated video-assisted thoracoscopic decortication in high-risk parapneumonic empyema patients. Surg Endosc 2017;31:1719–27.

35. Katlic MR, Facktor MA. Video-assisted thoracic surgery utilizing local anesthesia and sedation: 384 consecutive cases. Ann Thorac Surg 2010;90: 240–5.

36. Migliore M. Uniportal, single incision VATS for the skeptics. J Vis Surg 2018;4:97.

37. Migliore M. Uniportal video-assisted thoracic surgery: twentieth anniversary. J Thorac Dis 2018;10: 6442–5.

38. Cajozzo M, Lo Iacono G, Raffaele F, et al. Thoracoscopy in pleural effusion–two techniques: awake single-access video-assisted thoracic surgery versus 2-ports video-assisted thoracic surgery under general anesthesia. Future Oncol 2015; 11(24suppl):39–41.

39. Kiral H, Tezel C, Ocakcioglu I, et al. One-port videothoracoscopic surgical intervention. Surg Laparosc Endosc Percutan Tech 2015;25:40–2.

40. Hung MH, Hsu HH, Cheng YJ, et al. Nonintubated thoracoscopic surgery: state of the art and future directions. J Thorac Dis 2014;6:2.

41. Kara M, Alzafer S, Okur E, et al. The use of single incision thoracoscopic surgery in diagnostic and therapeutic thoracic surgical procedures. Acta Chir Belg 2013;113:25–9.

42. Pompeo E, Sorge R, Akopov A, et al, ESTS Non-intubated Thoracic Surgery Working Group. Non-intubated thoracic surgery—A survey from the European Society of Thoracic Surgeons. Ann Transl Med 2015;3:37.

43. Mineo TC, Tamburrini A, Perroni G, et al. 1000 cases of tubeless video-assisted thoracic surgery at the Rome Tor Vergata University. Future Oncol 2016; 12(23Suppl):13–8.

44. Tamburrini A, Mineo TC. A glimpse of history: non-intubated thoracic surgery. Video Assist Thorac Surg 2017;2:52.

Nonintubated Video-Assisted Thoracoscopic Surgery Lung Biopsy for Interstitial Lung Disease

Tae Ho Kim, MD, Jong Ho Cho, MD, PhD*

KEYWORDS

- Nonintubated surgery • Interstitial lung disease • Video-assisted thoracoscopic surgery (VATS)
- Wedge resection • Lung biopsy

KEY POINTS

- Thoracoscopic lung biopsy has been performed using a conventional positive-pressure ventilator under general anesthesia, but the complications associated with general anesthesia and positive-pressure ventilators are not negligible.
- Perioperative surgical outcomes for the nonintubated video-assisted thoracoscopic surgery (VATS) lung biopsy for interstitial lung disease are comparable with the intubated technique.
- Nonintubated VATS lung biopsy for interstitial lung disease is a safe and feasible option in carefully selected patients with interstitial lung disease.

INTRODUCTION

Interstitial lung diseases (ILDs) are a heterogeneous group with diffuse parenchymal lung disease. Although rare, they are classified with similar clinical, radiological, physiologic, or pathologic signs. Pathologic examination is required if clinical symptoms, blood tests, or high-resolution computed tomography (HRCT) images alone are not enough to diagnose ILD. This may be important because treatment options and prognosis differ greatly between the various types of ILD. Methods for pathologic examinations include transbronchial lung biopsy (TBLB) and surgical lung biopsy. Surgical lung biopsy is usually performed by video-assisted thoracoscopic surgery (VATS) under general anesthesia and provides excellent diagnostic results.[1,2] The diagnostic yield is up to 95% (range 85%–100%).[3]

Because most patients with ILD have impaired pulmonary function, the risks of thoracic surgery are an important issue when considering surgical lung biopsy. These morbidity and mortality rates are not negligible.

General thoracic surgery has evolved from a traditional open thoracotomy to VATS. VATS has been widely accepted because of its smaller incision, shorter hospital stays, and less pain and bleeding after surgery. General thoracic surgery is generally performed under general anesthesia and mechanical 1-lung ventilation owing to severe pain and cardiopulmonary physiologic change. Efforts have been made to prevent the complications following thoracic surgery caused by general anesthesia and the use of a positive-pressure ventilator.[4–7] The complications of general anesthesia and mechanical 1-lung ventilation are as follows. The ventilator-associated lung injury (more

Disclosure Statement: The authors have nothing to disclose.
Department of Thoracic and Cardiovascular Surgery, Samsung Medical Center, Sungkyunkwan University School of Medicine, 81 Irwon-ro, Gangnam-gu, Seoul 06351, Korea
* Corresponding author.
E-mail address: jongho.cho@gmail.com

Thorac Surg Clin 30 (2020) 41–48
https://doi.org/10.1016/j.thorsurg.2019.08.005
1547-4127/20/© 2019 Elsevier Inc. All rights reserved.

dangerous in patients with preexisting pulmonary disease) can be caused by positive-pressure ventilation. General anesthesia sometimes causes other complications, such as cardiac arrhythmia, transient hypoxemia, liver and kidney damage, impaired cognitive function, impaired preoperative immune surveillance, and mechanical airway injury.

Nonintubated VATS (NIVATS) is performed under spontaneous breathing and regional anesthesia without general anesthesia and positive-pressure mechanical ventilation. NIVATS was already introduced in the 1950s.[8] This method was not used for a long time but has begun to reappear as a way to reduce postoperative complications related to general anesthesia and mechanical ventilation. NIVATS is expanding from simple procedures (pleural effusion, pleural biopsy, pneumothorax, ILD wedge biopsy) to complex procedures (anatomic lung resections, thymectomy, sleeve lobectomy).[9–11] NIVATS may help achieve a shorter hospital stay and a reduction in postoperative morbidity rate compared with general anesthesia VATS in selected cases.[12]

NIVATS was particularly applied to people with poor cardiorespiratory function. Recently, adoption of NIVATS is being progressively extended to patients without any substantial risk factor for general anesthesia and 1-lung ventilation. Indeed, in a recent survey from the European Society of Thoracic Surgeons, 20% affirmed to favor to the use of NIVATS regardless of a patient's comorbidity profile.[13] However, simple procedures, such as pneumothorax and ILD lung biopsy, have a short operative time and not many complications. Therefore, the shortening of the hospital stay and the reduction of complications, which are known as the advantages of NIVATS, are not significant compared with general anesthesia VATS in these procedures. However, if a patient has impaired cardiopulmonary function, NIVATS can be applied to improve patient safety.

DIAGNOSIS

ILD is a generic term representing a heterogeneous group of diffuse parenchymal lung diseases classified together owing to several common features. The most common type of ILD is idiopathic pulmonary fibrosis (IPF). For diagnosis, a multidisciplinary team of experts is needed, which improves the accuracy of the diagnosis.[14] Both the clinical context given by the pulmonary clinician and interpretation of chest HRCT by thoracic radiologist are very important. If these are not enough to diagnose, additional information can

be obtained by bronchoalveolar lavage (BAL) and/or TBLB using bronchoscopy. Then, if the size of the specimen is not enough to diagnose, adequate large tissue should be obtained with surgical lung biopsy[15] (**Table 1**)

Clinical evaluation by the pulmonary clinician includes examining the patient's past medical history, physical examination, family history, and exposure to substances known to result in pulmonary injury. Clinical impression is obtained through various acquired clinical data. Image interpretation of the thoracic radiologist is crucial. HRCT chest scans are essential for ILD and should be taken with adequate inspiration and absent respiratory motion. Past chest imaging should be reviewed, and ILD can be narrowed down by combining these clinical and image data.

Because chest imaging is often seen in certain clinical situations, many disorders can be diagnosed with confidence without the need to obtain lung tissue. For example, in the case of a typical usual interstitial pneumonia (UIP) pattern on HRCT and a clinical context of idiopathic interstitial pneumonia (IIP), diagnosis of IPF does not require surgical lung biopsy. Connective tissue disease-associated ILD and ILD associated with a specific and clinically significant medication, environmental, occupational, avocational, or accidental exposure are also clinically diagnosed without pathologic lung tissue. However, if the imaging pattern is not typical within the clinical context, surgical lung biopsy should be considered (**Fig. 1**).

INDICATIONS

TBLB can be safely obtained by flexible bronchoscopy. Specimens by TBLB are a few millimeters in size. The biopsy forceps passes through the pathway of the bronchoscope. TBLB is often chosen when the suspected ILD is centrilobularly located. Examples of such diseases include sarcoidosis, hypersensitivity pneumonitis, lymphangitic carcinomatosis, eosinophilic pneumonia, infections, and alveolar proteinosis.[16,17] However, TBLB is less likely to be helpful if the pattern of HRCT is uncertain or indicates IIP. TBLB cannot be used to diagnose IPF because it cannot adequately diagnose UIP associated with IPF. BAL cell differential counts can differentiate diseases such as eosinophilic pneumonia.

SURGICAL LUNG BIOPSY

Surgical lung biopsy is performed when a larger specimen is needed for diagnosis than a TBLB.

Table 1
Nonintubated video-assisted thoracoscopic surgery lung biopsy for interstitial lung disease

Author, Year	Subjects (n)	Context	Analgesia	Sedation Level	Wedge Number	Operative Time	Conversion to General Anesthesia	Diagnosis	Morbidity and Mortality	Observation Period
Ambrogi & Mineo,[29] 2014	40	3-port (20) 1-port (20)	TEA (20) ICB (20)	Mild (midazolam or propofol)	2.3 2.1	38 40	1 (5%) 1 (5%)	33 (82.5%)	ARDS (1) Pneumonia (1)	2002–2014
Peng et al,[28] 2017	43	1-port tubeless LMA (SIMV)	IV analgesia	BIS 40–60	2	22 ± 5	0[a]	38 (88.4%)	Atrial fibrillation (1) Pneumonia (1) Chest tube insertion (1)	2014–2015
Jeon et al,[19] 2018	10	3-port Facial mask	TEA	BIS 60–80	2	33	0	10 (100%)	0	2016

Abbreviations: ARDS, acute respiratory distress syndrome; BIS, bispectral index; ICB, intercostal block; IV, intravenous; LMA, laryngeal mask airway; SIMV, synchronized intermittent mandatory ventilation; TEA, thoracic epidural anesthesia
[a] Conversion to 2-port and chest tube or urinary catheterization in 3 cases.

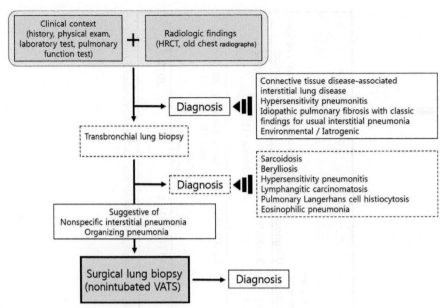

Fig. 1. Schematic of surgical lung biopsy for ILD.

Specimens can be obtained by VATS or open thoracotomy. Diagnostic yields are reported in the range of 85% to 100%.[3,18,19] There are various opinions on the appropriate volume and number of specimens in ILD surgical biopsy. Ideally, biopsies are obtained from multiple lobes with varying severity because studies suggest this improves diagnostic accuracy.[20] Guidelines suggest that more than 1 specimen should be collected when biopsy is performed.[21,22] After careful examination via HRCT, the location of the wedge resection is decided by considering the extent and distribution of the lesion. When the wedge resection is performed, the lesion is resected to a size sufficient to include some of the healthy tissue. To provide the pathologist with the appropriate tissue to assess the pattern and distribution of the disease, the lung biopsy sample should be larger than 4 cm in the greatest dimension when inflated and include a width of 3 cm to 5 cm.[16]

The morbidity and mortality of surgical lung biopsy are not negligible because most patients with ILD have impaired pulmonary function. After the procedure, the 30-day mortality rate varies from 0% to 24%, according to several reports.[1,23] Another study reported that surgical lung biopsies for ILD from hospitals across the United States had an in-hospital mortality of just under 2% for elective operations but a significantly increased mortality (16%) for nonelective (urgent and emergency) procedures.[24] Patients with an acute exacerbation of their ILD at the time of biopsy are at a high risk of postoperative complications and death. However, these postoperative deaths should be interpreted in the context of the high mortality rate of patients with IPF worsening without surgical lung biopsy.

Previously, when surgical lung biopsy was needed in patients with impaired pulmonary function, open thoracotomy was preferred because 1-lung ventilation was not required. Currently, tissue can be obtained without 1-lung ventilation via NIVATS. NIVATS is performed under spontaneous breathing and regional anesthesia, without general anesthesia and positive-pressure mechanical ventilation. Recently, adoption of NIVATS is being progressively extended to patients without any substantial risk factors for general anesthesia and 1-lung ventilation.

TECHNICAL FEASIBILITY

NIVATS lung biopsy has several important differences from surgery under general anesthesia and with a positive-pressure ventilator. It does not use a double-lumen endotracheal tube so airway injury can be avoided. It is possible to reduce the risk of ventilator-induced lung injury due to negative-pressure ventilation by maintaining the patient's spontaneous respiration without giving positive pressure using mechanical ventilation. Also, muscle relaxants are not used because the patient's spontaneous breathing must be maintained.

THE PROCEDURE UNDER GENERAL ANESTHESIA

The detailed techniques used in the authors' center are as follows, starting with a brief introduction to the typical VATS procedure under general anesthesia with 1-lung ventilation usually performed at the hospital. In the operating room, the standard monitoring devices, including electrocardiography, pulse oximeter, end-tidal carbon dioxide ($ETCO_2$), and bispectral index (BIS) were applied. Endotracheal intubation was performed via the routine double-lumen endotracheal intubation procedure using muscle relaxants and sedatives. An arterial catheter was placed in the radial artery opposite the surgical site for invasive arterial blood pressure monitoring. The patient's posture was changed from the supine to the lateral decubitus position, with the surgical site upwards. A 10.5-mm or 5.5-mm camera port and a 5.5-mm instrumentation port were inserted. Pleural exploration, thorough valuation for pleura and lung surface, was performed. An additional 12-mm port was made for using the endoscopic stapler. One or 2 sites of wedge resections were performed with Endo GIA 60-4.8mm (Medtronic, Minneapolis, USA) endoscopic staplers. After the operation, 1 12F or 20F chest tube was placed via the VATS port.

In NIVATS cases, difficulty in breathing may be caused by hypoxia, insufficient pain management, or sedation. Generally, inspiratory oxygen can be increased as a first maneuver for correction. In the case of insufficient pain management or sedation, additional anesthetic medications may be required. The use of dexmedetomidine for patients with severe respiratory dysfunction might be preferable during NIVATS. If these treatments are not enough to stabilize the patient's hemodynamics, the conversion to general anesthesia by intubation should be considered.

NONINTUBATED (AWAKE) PROCEDURE

NIVATS differs in many ways from the conventional procedure. Among the many types of locoregional anesthesia to reduce pain, the authors used epidural anesthesia for NIVATS. Some other groups used intercostal blocks or only local anesthesia. Thoracic epidural catheterization was performed by an anesthesiologist from the pain service team on the same day of the surgery. With the patient in a prone position and under the guidance of fluoroscopy, a 19-gauge epidural catheter, FlexTipPlus (Arrow International, Morrisville, USA) was inserted into the thoracic nerve T6 to T7 intervertebral space and the catheter tip was advanced up to T5. The position of the epidural catheter tip was confirmed by dispersion of a contrast medium. An epidural test dose of 3 mL was then performed, comprising 1.5% lidocaine and 15 μg epinephrine.

In the operating room, the standard monitoring devices, including electrocardiography, pulse oximeter, $ETCO_2$, and BIS were applied. This process is the same as the intubated procedure. Lidocaine nebulization of 4 mL at 4% concentration using the Nebulizer (PARI, Moosstrasse 3, Germany) was administered for 15 minutes to suppress coughing. A cannula was inserted into the radial artery for invasive arterial blood pressure monitoring while the patient was on lidocaine nebulization. Drug injection for thoracic blockade was started. Ropivacaine (15 mL at 0.75%) mixed with fentanyl (1 mL of 50 μg) was administered for the thoracic blockade. A T3 to T10 sensory block was planned to enable multiport surgery and chest tube insertion. Local anesthetic (3–4 mL) was administered incrementally through the epidural catheter after catheter aspiration. A dermatomal block was confirmed using warm-cold discrimination. Prepared local anesthetics (14 mL) were administered to reach the T3 sensory block within 15 minutes. A final check of the sensory block before surgery confirmed coverage from T2 to T11. After 20 minutes, the remaining 2 mL of prepared local anesthetic was administered through the epidural catheter to maintain anesthesia.[25]

Conscious sedation was maintained during operation with a remifentanil (0.0–0.5 μg/kg/min) or dexmedetomidine (0.3–0.5 μg/kg/h) infusion and the dose was titrated to maintain a BIS of 60 to 80 during surgery. Oxygen (5 L/min at 100% concentration) was administered via a facial mask, with an $ETCO_2$ monitoring line attached to the mask during surgery. In case of low saturation (<95%), the oxygen fraction of facial mask was increased and patient was encouraged to breathe deeply. An endotracheal tube; a fiberoptic bronchoscope; a supraglottic airway, i-gel (Intersurgical Ltd, Wokingham, United Kingdom); and a bronchial blocker were prepared in the operating room for emergent conversion to general anesthesia.

The patient's posture was changed from the supine to the lateral decubitus position, with the surgical site upwards. We used the same utility port of single-incision laparoscopic surgery for NIVATS biopsy to decrease patient discomfort and achieve better control of collapse and inflation of the operated lung. This was also effective in reducing coughing by minimizing pleural irritations, which can be caused by airflow. The operation started with 4 cm of skin incision on the (usually) 5th intercostal space after enough skin and subcutaneous tissue local infiltration. The 4-cm uniport utility, Glove Port 4220-AS-3 (Nelis Medical, Bucheon, Korea), was then inserted (**Fig. 2**). At the time the scope was inserted, the lung became atelectatic within first 10 minutes. The lung remained atelectatic until the end of the operation. The surgical lung biopsies were performed by 1 or 2 wedge resections of lung regions deemed radiologically and macroscopically more representative for diagnosis using standard method. Intraoperative vagal nerve block or phrenic nerve block was not required because only simple wedge resection was performed. At the end of the procedure, 1 12F or 20F chest tube was left in situ. The patient was transferred to the postanesthesia care unit after changing to the supine position after surgery.

During the surgery, the patient was awake and the operation time was short so urinary catheterization was usually not required. In some elderly male patients with symptomatic benign prostatic hyperplasia, epidural anesthesia could induce severe urinary retention, so

urinary catheterization was required in selected patients.

POSTOPERATIVE CARE

The patient was transferred to the general ward through the postanesthesia care unit after surgery. All patients were evaluated via chest radiography every day. Chest tube removal was performed if chest tube drainage was less than 200 mL for 24 hours with sufficient lung recruitment and no air leakage on chest radiography. The patient was discharged the next day after a chest tube removal if there was no specific medical problem. Two weeks after discharge, the patient visited the outpatient clinic where wound and chest radiographs were examined.

OPERATIVE OUTCOMES

Regardless of the type and extent of surgery, a meta-analysis review article on NIVATS has been reported.[12,26] Also, the results of ILD biopsy using general anesthesia VATS have been reported for a long time.[27] However, there are few reports of biopsy operations for the diagnosis of ILD in NIVATS (see **Table 1**).[19,28,29] The number of ports was not significantly influenced by the operation performed in a short time. Thoracic epidural anesthesia or intercostal blocks (ICBs) were mainly used for pain control. Comparing the 2 methods, there is a report that an ICB is a benefit in operation time and hospital stay.[29,30] In most surgeries, an average of 2 tissues were obtained and the diagnostic rate was 82.5% to 100%. The operation time is generally short, from 22 to 40 minutes. There was no in-hospital mortality. NIVATS biopsy resulted in low morbidity (3.3%–7.0%).

SUMMARY

The perioperative surgical outcomes for the nonintubated VATS lung biopsy for ILD are comparable to the intubated technique. NIVATS lung biopsy (especially in ILD) may be safe and feasible option in patients with poor lung function for whom general anesthesia is contraindicated. Importantly, these preliminary results have to be confirmed by a larger study to assess the long-term effects and diagnostic rate of this less-invasive surgical strategy.

REFERENCES

1. Lee YC, Wu CT, Hsu HH, et al. Surgical lung biopsy for diffuse pulmonary disease: experience of 196

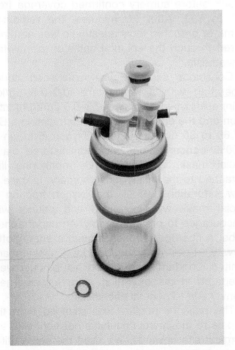

Fig. 2. Glove port 4220-AS-3. (*Courtesy of* Nelis Medical, Bucheon, Korea.)

patients. J Thorac Cardiovasc Surg 2005;129: 984–90.

2. Zhang D, Liu Y. Surgical lung biopsies in 418 patients with suspected interstitial lung disease in China. Intern Med 2010;49:1097–102.

3. Han Q, Luo Q, Xie JX, et al. Diagnostic yield and postoperative mortality associated with surgical lung biopsy for evaluation of interstitial lung diseases: A systematic review and meta-analysis. J Thorac Cardiovasc Surg 2015;149: 1394–1401 e1.

4. Slutsky AS. History of mechanical ventilation. From Vesalius to ventilator-induced lung injury. Am J Respir Crit Care Med 2015;191:1106–15.

5. Zochios V, Hague M, Giraud K, et al. Lung protective mechanical ventilation strategies in cardiothoracic critical care: a retrospective study. Int J Gen Med 2016;9:415–8.

6. Amar D, Zhang H, Pedoto A, et al. Protective lung ventilation and morbidity after pulmonary resection: a propensity score-matched analysis. Anesth Analg 2017;125:190–9.

7. Kim HJ, Cha SI, Kim CH, et al. Risk factors of postoperative acute lung injury following lobectomy for nonsmall cell lung cancer. Medicine (Baltimore) 2019;98(13):e15078.

8. Buckingham WW, Beatty AJ, Brasher CA, et al. The technique of administering epidural anesthesia in thoracic surgery. Dis Chest 1950;17:561–8.

9. Herrmann D, Volmerig J, Hecker E. Non-intubated uniportal video-assisted thoracoscopic surgery for carinal sleeve resection-is surgical process almost completed? J Thorac Dis 2018; 10:145–7.

10. Gonzalez-Rivas D, Bonome C, Fieira E, et al. Non-intubated video-assisted thoracoscopic lung resections: the future of thoracic surgery? Eur J Cardiothorac Surg 2016;49:721–31.

11. Matsumoto I, Oda M, Watanabe G. Awake endoscopic thymectomy via an infrasternal approach using sternal lifting. Thorac Cardiovasc Surg 2008;56: 311–3.

12. Tacconi F, Pompeo E. Non-intubated video-assisted thoracic surgery: where does evidence stand? J Thorac Dis 2016;8:S364–75.

13. Pompeo E, Sorge R, Akopov A, et al. Non-intubated thoracic surgery - A survey from the European Society of Thoracic Surgeons. Ann Transl Med 2015;3:37.

14. Flaherty KR, King TE Jr, Raghu G, et al. Idiopathic interstitial pneumonia: what is the effect of a multidisciplinary approach to diagnosis? Am J Respir Crit Care Med 2004;170:904–10.

15. Raj R, Raparia K, Lynch DA, et al. Surgical lung biopsy for interstitial lung diseases. Chest 2017;151: 1131–40.

16. Bradley B, Branley HM, Egan JJ, et al. Interstitial lung disease guideline: the British Thoracic Society in collaboration with the Thoracic Society of Australia and New Zealand and the Irish Thoracic Society. Thorax 2008;63(Suppl 5):v1–58.

17. Ensminger SA, Prakash UB. Is bronchoscopic lung biopsy helpful in the management of patients with diffuse lung disease? Eur Respir J 2006;28: 1081–4.

18. Morell F, Reyes L, Domenech G, et al. Diagnoses and diagnostic procedures in 500 consecutive patients with clinical suspicion of interstitial lung disease. Arch Bronconeumol 2008;44: 185–91.

19. Jeon CS, Yoon DW, Moon SM, et al. Non-intubated video-assisted thoracoscopic lung biopsy for interstitial lung disease: a single-center experience. J Thorac Dis 2018;10:3262–8.

20. Flint A, Martinez FJ, Young ML, et al. Influence of sample number and biopsy site on the histologic diagnosis of diffuse lung disease. Ann Thorac Surg 1995;60:1605–7.

21. Raghu G, Remy-Jardin M, Myers JL, et al. Diagnosis of idiopathic pulmonary fibrosis. An official ATS/ERS/JRS/ALAT clinical practice guideline. Am J Respir Crit Care Med 2018;198:e44–68.

22. Fibla JJ, Brunelli A, Allen MS, et al. Do the number and volume of surgical lung biopsies influence the diagnostic yield in interstitial lung disease? a propensity score analysis. Arch Bronconeumol 2015; 51:76–9.

23. Plones T, Osei-Agyemang T, Elze M, et al. Morbidity and mortality in patients with usual interstitial pneumonia (UIP) pattern undergoing surgery for lung biopsy. Respir Med 2013;107:629–32.

24. Hutchinson JP, Fogarty AW, McKeever TM, et al. In-hospital mortality after surgical lung biopsy for Interstitial Lung Disease in the United States. 2000 to 2011. Am J Respir Crit Care Med 2016; 193:1161–7.

25. Kim KY, Lee GH, Cho JH, et al. Non-intubated video-assisted thoracoscopic biopsy surgery of a large anterior mediastinal mass via epidural anesthesia -A case report. Anesthesiol Pain Med 2017;12: 256–60.

26. Fibla JJ, Molins L, Blanco A, et al. Video-assisted thoracoscopic lung biopsy in the diagnosis of interstitial lung disease: a prospective, multi-center study in 224 patients. Arch Bronconeumol 2012; 48:81–5.

27. Morris D, Zamvar V. The efficacy of video-assisted thoracoscopic surgery lung biopsies in patients with Interstitial Lung Disease: a retrospective study of 66 patients. J Cardiothorac Surg 2014;9:45.

28. Peng G, Liu M, Luo Q, et al. Spontaneous ventilation anesthesia combined with uniportal and tubeless

thoracoscopic lung biopsy in selected patients with interstitial lung diseases. J Thorac Dis 2017;9: 4494–501.

29. Ambrogi V, Mineo TC. VATS biopsy for undetermined interstitial lung disease under non-general anesthesia: comparison between uniportal

approach under intercostal block vs. three-ports in epidural anesthesia. J Thorac Dis 2014;6: 888–95.

30. Pompeo E, Rogliani P, Cristino B, et al. Awake thoracoscopic biopsy of interstitial lung disease. Ann Thorac Surg 2013;95:445–52.

Nonintubated Video-Assisted Wedge Resections in Peripheral Lung Cancer

Vincenzo Ambrogi, MD, PhD[a,b,*], Riccardo Tajè, MS[b],
Tommaso Claudio Mineo, MD[a,†]

KEYWORDS

- Lung cancer • VATS • Nonintubated thoracic surgery

KEY POINTS

- Wedge resection in lung cancer is considered a suboptimal procedure, but in elderly and/or frail patients is a reliable and safer alternative.
- Nonintubated thoracic surgery may allow reduction of operative time, postoperative morbidity, hospital stay, and global economical expenses.
- Nonintubated modality can allow the recruitment of patients considered otherwise marginal for a surgical treatment.
- The nonintubated video-assisted thoracic surgery approach is less traumatic, with less immunologic impairment, which may affect postoperative oncological long-term results.

INTRODUCTION

Since the beginning of the nonintubated program, the resection of peripheral undetermined pulmonary nodules was generally believed to be among the main indications for procedures under this kind of anesthesia.[1] Within this group of operations, surgeons have also resected a significant number of lesions that resulted from primitive early and peripheral lung cancer. Unfortunately, limited resection of lung cancer is still considered suboptimal from the oncological point of view and this argument has considerably restricted the indications for nonintubated surgery of lung cancer. Conversely, this anesthetic modality extended the indications for surgery to even the most fragile and oldest patients.[2] Thus, this type of surgery has grown in the space allowed between these 2 extremes: questionable radicality and great tolerability. This article describes the various nonintubated video-assisted thoracic surgery (VATS) techniques for resection of peripheral lung cancer and tries to individuate the main indications for this kind of surgery that, in the authors' opinions, deserves a particular and precise space in the armamentarium of a thoracic surgeon.

ANESTHESIA

At first, surgeons performed procedures under thoracic epidural anesthesia (TEA), which could simultaneously cover 3 or 4 metameric regions and allowed a triportal access.[3]

TEA is usually established at the thoracic nerve–4 level by the insertion of an epidural catheter to maintain a continuous infusion of 1.66 µg/mL sufentanil and 0.5% ropivacaine. If the somatosensory block is insufficient, a supplement of

Disclosure: The authors have nothing to disclose.
[a] Department of Surgical Sciences, Tor Vergata University, Via Montpellier 1, Rome 00133, Italy; [b] Division of Thoracic Surgery, Tor Vergata University Policlinic, Viale Oxford 81, Rome 00133, Italy
[†] Deceased.
* Corresponding author. Department of Surgical Sciences, Tor Vergata University, Via Montpellier 1, Rome 00133, Italy.
E-mail address: ambrogi@med.uniroma2.it

Thorac Surg Clin 30 (2020) 49–59
https://doi.org/10.1016/j.thorsurg.2019.08.006

7.5% ropivacaine and 2% bupivacaine can be added at incision sites.[4] Atropine (0.01 mg/kg) or 5 mL of aerosolized 2% lidocaine can be used to reduce the cough reflex. However, these drugs are more likely to be superfluous because the peripheral maneuvering of the lung parenchyma does not produce high stimulation to the vagus nerve.[5,6]

The reduction of surgical incisions allowed the shift from TEA to local anesthesia. To obtain an adequate analgesia, we separately inject lidocaine 2% (4 mg/kg) at the site of incision and up to the parietal pleura, and 7.5% ropivacaine (2 mg/kg) along the competent intercostal nerve (**Fig. 1**).

Meanwhile, anesthesiologists refined protocols and techniques, taking advantage of the newest technology, such as bispectral index (BIS) monitoring and vagal blockade.[7] In particular, the introduction of BIS allowed a better control of drug delivery during procedure. Anesthesia can be conducted by keeping the BIS index around 90 to 100,[8] or with a light to moderate sedation (60–90) for patients who are more anxious.

Finally, it must be remembered that these patients are usually sensitive about the impact of the diagnosis on their lives, and this feeling may considerably increase during the procedure. For this reason, a deeper sedation can be

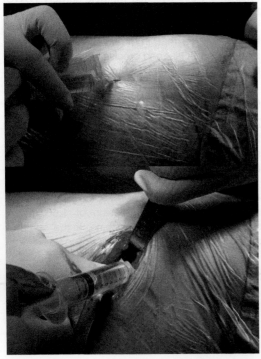

Fig. 1. Skin infiltration with local anesthetic on the site of the incision (*top*), intercostal nerve blockade after skin incision (*bottom*).

useful when resection becomes unexpectedly demanding. An intravenous dose of propofol (10 mg/mL) can be injected and maintained using a target-controlled infusion with a progressive supplement of fentanyl.[9,10]

SURGERY

It must be stressed that the atmosphere of the operating room deserves particular attention. It must be kept quiet and professional. All personnel should be well-trained and should avoid direct comments about the pathologic condition, as well as agitated status or inopportune noise. Extensive use of low-volume, calm, and relaxing music can help.

Technological progress and experience has allowed surgeons to enrich their repertoire of techniques. This article describes the classic triportal, biportal, and uniportal approaches that the authors have experience with.

Patient Selection

A patient being considered for nonintubated VATS wedge resections should have several characteristics. First, the features of the mass should be suitable for a quick wedge resection with an adequate resection margin free of tumor. In order to fit this mandatory prerequisite, 2 critical parameters should be taken into account: the diameter and location of the nodule. Generally, the maximal permitted diameter should not exceed 3 cm[11]; however, in the case of a safe nonintubated wedge, the authors recommend a much smaller size. In our opinion, this critical limit should be set to 2 cm, but we assume that the smaller the size results in easier and safer resection (**Fig. 2**).

The mass should be peripherally located preferably no deeper than 1 cm from the external visceral pleura, or in alternative adjacent to the external margin of a fissure. Mass located in the fissure should be superficial and far from the pulmonary artery branches. Another demanding location for a nonintubated wedge resection is the basal surface of the lower lobes, which can become particularly problematic when the nodule is located in proximity to the inferior pulmonary vein. To better evaluate the exact distance from the nearest fissure, it may be helpful to visualize the nodule on computed tomography (CT) scan, according to sagittal and coronal planes. **Fig. 3** shows a polyaxial map of the lung regions where a nodule can lie to be considered feasible for a nonintubated wedge resection.

Notwithstanding, the presence of pliable emphysematous tissue should allow the resection of a deeply located and otherwise unresectable

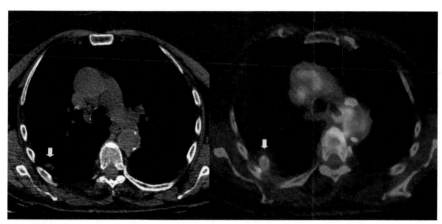

Fig. 2. Chest CT (*left*) and PET (*right*) scan showing the same pulmonary nodule (*arrows*) of the superior segment of the right lower lobe feasible for nonintubated VATS wedge resection.

nodule, especially if located in the apical regions of the lobes. Another major contraindication to neoplastic, radical, nonintubated wedge resection is imaging evidence of enlarged or clearly neoplastic mediastinal lymph nodes. In these conditions, the use of CT scan combined with PET can be of great use. Nevertheless, diagnostic resections are progressively gaining importance and will be a topic of future discussion.

Obviously, one should also consider general contraindications to nonintubated anesthesia, which are summarized in **Box 1**.[5]

Patient Position

An important premise to remember for patient position is that the surgeon is operating on an awake patient; therefore, he or she must acquire and keep a very comfortable position for the duration of the procedure. As for surgery under general anesthesia and 1-lung ventilation, the patient should usually lie on lateral decubitus. If tolerable, the table should be flexed at the level of the nipple to allow a better exposure of the intercostal spaces (**Fig. 4**). Similtaneouly, to decrease tension on the upside hip, a pillow can be placed between the legs. Some centers insert an additional bed sheet under the back of the patient to allow rapid change of position in the case of urgent intubation. However, in the event of nodule sited in the most anterior region of the lobes, the procedure may be performed in a semisupine position through a uniportal approach similar to that adopted in cases of thymectomy.[12]

Surgeon and Equipment Positions

In the authors' experience, the surgeon preferably stands facing the patient. The first assistant stands on the opposite side of the surgeon and, if a second assistant is available, he or she holds the camera standing caudally to the surgeon. The scrub nurse stands sideways to the first assistant. The main video monitor and the anesthesiologist occupy a position above the head of the patient. The suction devices and the electrocautery and energy tools are placed at the side of the operating table. A water seal system should be always kept ready on the instrument table.

Armamentarium

All the instruments are common to those used for VATS, such as a 30-degree thoracoscope, endoclamps, endostaplers, endoclip appliers, and the energy devices, either radiofrequency or ultrasound. New dedicated instruments are indispensabile for uniportal access. These tools are usually long, narrow-shafted, bent, and double-hinged.

In cases of urgent intubation, the anesthesiologist should have ready a double-lumen tube, laryngeal mask, fiberoptic bronchoscope with a video-assisted system, and an endobronchial blocker to safely assess the most suitable device according to the situation.[6]

Classic Triportal Surgery

The classic triportal approach was the first access introduced for nonintubated video-assisted wedge resections in peripheral lung cancer.[4] Due to the multilocation of the ports, this approach should be accomplished under TEA that can simultaneously cover the 3 or 4 metameric regions involved in the procedure.

The authors place the 3 ports following the so-called baseball-diamond setting, with the camera in the center as the homebase, pointing to the lesion as the second base, and with the remaining 2 operative ports placed as first and third bases, respectively (**Fig. 5**).

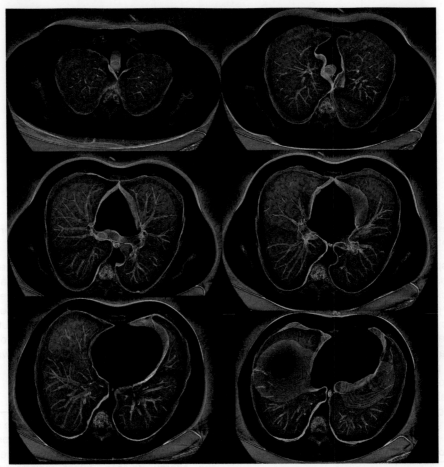

Fig. 3. Polyaxial CT thick scans with chromatic elaboration evident at different levels the areas (*pink*) suitable for nonintubated VATS resection of nodules. Apical regions (*upper left and right*), carena level (*middle left*), pulmonary veins level (*middle right*), middle lobe and lingular basal regions (*lower left*) and lower lobes basal regions (*lower right*).

The first port is generally created at the 4th or 5th intercostal space on the anterior axillary line. A wise strategy is to first insert the 30-degree camera and, from this access, to visualize all the following ports. At this level, the intercostal space is wider and this minimizes trauma to the underlying nerves.[5] The second port is placed at the 7th intercostal space on the anterior axillary line. This is the camera port where the pleural drainage tube will be placed at the end of the procedure. The last port is positioned on the posterior axillary line, again at the 4th or 5th intercostal space.

Three ports can be very useful at the beginning of the learning curve because they can control the respiratory movement of the breathing lung through a surgical instrument.[9]

Digital exploration can be usually made through the port closer to the lesion, which can be conveniently enlarged if required. Generally, the observation of visceral pleural retraction or scarring can reveal malignant lesions. After having identified the lesion, it can be excised by staplers. It could be helpful to previously circumscribe the nodule with a vascular clamp, tracing the pathway for the stapler and facilitating its insertion. Once the stapler is applied, a good habit can be to repalpate the nodule in order to ensure its presence and appreciate the consistency of the resection margin before the excision. The excised nodule and the adjacent parenchyma is preferably placed in a retrieval bag and extracted from the most anterior and larger port. The specimen is always oriented to recognize visceral or stapling margins, and accurately inspected to confirm the successful and adequate resection of the lesion. Finally, hemostasis is visually ensured and any fluid collected in the pleural cavity is then removed. All the incisions, except the lowest where the chest tube should be placed under visual control, are closed in layers.

Box 1
General contraindications to nonintubated anesthesia

VATS feasibility

  Anamnestic or imaging absence of pleural adhesion

  No previous homolateral thoracoscopic surgery

  Normal coagulation tests and absence of bleeding disorders

  Nonobesity (body mass index <30 kg/m^2)

Nonintubated procedure feasibility

  Signed, fully informed consent to awake nonintubated procedure

  Easy accessibility to the airways

  Stable and cooperative psychological profile

  American Society of Anesthesiologists Physical Status Classification lower than III

  Presence of comorbidity

TEA feasibility

  Low risk of intraoperative seizure

  Absence of brain edema

  No spine deformities

  No coagulopathy

  Hemodynamic stability

Local anesthesia feasibility

  No history of allergy to local anesthesia

  Short-length of procedure

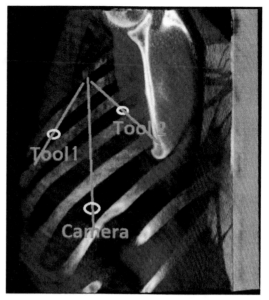

Fig. 5. Triportal scheme indicating camera and tools position.

Biportal Video-Assisted Thoracic Surgery

Discomfort during the procedure and postoperative pain have been proved to be minimized by the limitation of the number of surgical incisions.[9] Following the technical innovation in VATS under general anesthesia, we also try to avoid the posterior port in awake surgery. This expedient was very useful in the shift from TEA to local anesthesia with intravenous sedation.

The trocar disposition is quite similar to that of the triportal. The camera port is placed at the 7th intercostal place on the anterior axillary line and a wider operative port is placed at the 4th or 5th intercostal space on the same line (**Fig. 6**). Considerable aid is provided with the introduction of an annular sleeve-shaped self-retractor inserted in the anterior space. In fact, this tool makes it possible to achieve adequate surgical retraction and palpation using a wider utility port.

During the procedure, the position of the thoracoscope and mechanical stapler can be interchanged as needed to facilitate exposure of all visual angles and manipulation of the parenchyma (**Fig. 7**).

When the nodule is identified, the visceral surface of the lung is grasped with a forceps, and the endostapler is applied beneath the elevated lung tissue deep to the subpleural lesion. Often, the most suitable angle is achieved with introduction of the stapling device through the most inferior port (**Fig. 8**). Before firing, the staple line is inspected from both sides, and then the

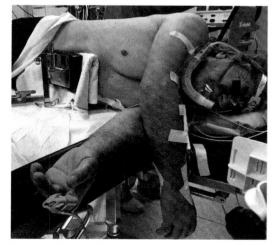

Fig. 4. Patient position for right-sided uniportal nonintubated VATS wedge resection.

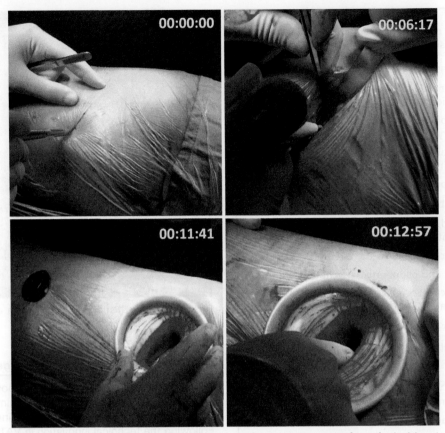

Fig. 6. Right biportal nonintubated VATS wedge resection with partial time spent from the incision. Incision (*upper left*), opening of the pleural space (*upper right*), protection of the utility port and the videoport with the annular retractor (*lower left*), and palpation through the utility port (*lower right*).

parenchyma can be resected. After completion of the resection, the lung is inspected for adequate hemostasis and pneumostasis. As previously described for the triportal approach, the specimen is retrieved into an endoscopic specimen bag to avoid incidental parietal seeding. A chest tube is positioned under visual control through the camera port toward a posterior apical position and reexpansion. The operative port is sutured in layers, avoiding intercostal stitching.

Uniportal Video-Assisted Thoracic Surgery

Nonintubated uniportal VATS technique has been used in most of the thoracic procedures, from minor to major surgery.[7] Therefore, it is natural to also extend it to wedge resections. Uniportal VATS has been proved to attenuate postoperative pain, residual paresthesia, and hospitalization compared with multiportal VATS.[13] Moreover, patients are usually more amenable to undergoing surgical procedures for early diagnosis and treatment of indeterminate lung nodules when a minimalistic approach is proposed.[14]

The introduction of the intraoperative vagal block made reduction of respiratory movements possible, facilitating this approach. Another refinement was achieved with the development of specifically designed thoracoscopic instruments, thus reducing the conflict and visualization problems related the forced point-of-view related to a unique port.[9] Under local anesthesia, a single operative port of 3 cm can be made at the 5th intercostal space along the anterior axillary line. Once the lung collapsed due to the iatrogenic pneumothorax, the working port should be protected by a plastic sleeve-shaped retractor (**Fig. 9**).

Exploration of the pleural cavity can be done through a 30-degree video thoracoscope, which is always placed at the most posterior end of the incision. A vagal nerve blockade can be performed to reduce the coughing reflex during lung manipulations. Injection of 3 mL of bupivacaine into the vagus nerve near the lower paratracheal (for right-sided procedures) and the aortopulmonary window (for left-sided procedures) can be performed.[15]

To attenuate the impact of intraoperative mediastinal oscillation, breathing frequency, and tidal

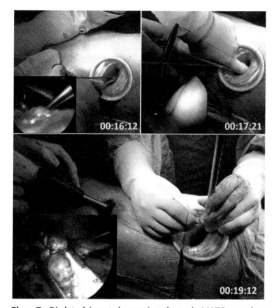

Fig. 7. Right biportal nonintubated VATS wedge resection with partial time spent from the skin incision. External and internal (*insets*) views. Stitching of the detected nodule (*upper left*), repalpation of the detected nodule (*upper right*), and positioning of the first stapler line (*bottom*).

volume during surgery, the anesthesiologist can also increase the amount of remifentanil (0.04 µg/kg/min). Similataneously, appropriate ventilation should be provided according to the results of blood gas analysis to avoid severe hypercapnia and to maintain the body's acid–base balance.[16]

The nodule can be localized, by direct vision, instrumental palpation, or other strategies (**Fig. 10**) as subsequently described in the dedicated paragraph.

When the site of the lesion is assessed, a forceps or 2 or more 2-0 silk anchoring retraction sutures can be used to suspend the lesion and the stapler insertion. A vascular clamp can be positioned under, proximal to the nodule, to reduce the burden of tissue between the stapler jaws facilitating the bite entry (see **Fig. 10**). The resected specimen can be removed with an endoscopic retrieval bag (**Fig. 11**) and should be examined in order to assess the success of the resection and the oncological radicality. Hemostasis and pneumostasis are visually ensured, and a chest tube (28F) can be placed under visual control toward the posterior apical position. The incision should be closed in layers. The level of the unique port affects the placement of the chest tube, which is sometimes too cephalic to adequately drain the

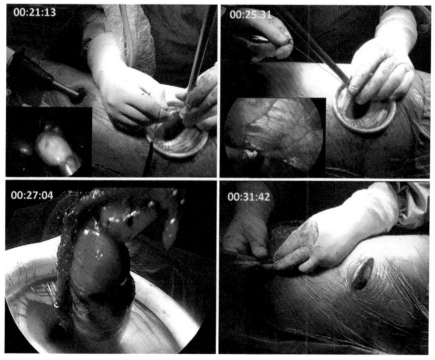

Fig. 8. Right biportal nonintubated VATS wedge resection with partial time spent from the incision. First stapling line firing (*upper left*), second and last stapling line firing (*upper right*), specimen extraction (*lower left*), and chest tube positioning (*lower right*).

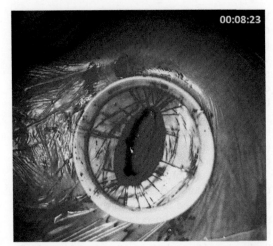

Fig. 9. Right uniportal nonintubated VATS wedge resection view with partial time spent from the skin incision. The port is protected by a sleeve plastic self-retractor.

posterior costophrenic sinus. For this reason, pleural liquid can accumulate below the level of the thoracostomy, hindering lung reexpansion and causing infection. To avoid this inconvenience, the chest tube should follow a J-shaped

pathway or, alternatively, a double-coaxial fenestrated lumen chest drain could be used. We found that the insertion of a 24F T-tube similar to that used in biliary tract surgery is helpful (**Fig. 12**). This tube is long and large enough to allow proper evacuation of both fluid and air. It is less painful compared with a larger tube and it is easily extracted from a uniportal incision.

Nodule Detection

Nodule detection can be challenging, even if the patient has been accurately selected and the anatomy of the lesion has been previously assessed. Thus, several techniques have been evaluated to ease this first step of the procedure. Intraoperative ultrasounds, dye tracers, or preoperative needle localization have been described[17]; however, in the authors' experience, digital palpation is effective enough. If the sole methodical digital palpation is not successful, better results can be achieved through a preoperative assessment of radiological landmarks, such as the distance separating the closest fissure and the nodule, and instrumental palpation can be accomplished by sliding the parenchyma with a ring-forceps. Nonetheless, if the lesion is still undetectable, it could be

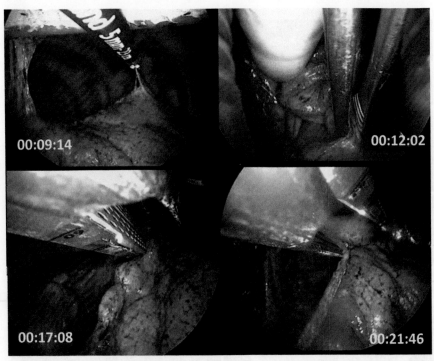

Fig. 10. Right uniportal nonintubated VATS wedge resection view with partial time spent from the skin incision. Videothoracoscopic views. Resection with energy device of pleuropulmonary adherences (*upper left*), palpation of the lesion sited in the upperlobe (*upper right*), first stapling firing (*lower left*), and second stapling firing (*lower right*).

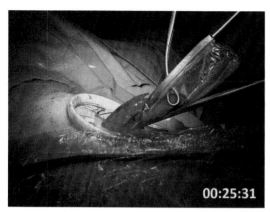

Fig. 11. Right uniportal nonintubated VATS wedge resection view with partial time spent from the skin incision. The lesion is extracted with an endobag.

advantageous to extend the anterior end of the surgical wound, taking advantage of the wider anterior intercostal space. Obviously, the enlargement of the operative field should be preceded by infiltration of the area with local anesthesia.

Resection

As previously stated, resections that are too demanding should be avoided. The use of the appropriate stapler bite is very important and much depends on the surgeon's preference.

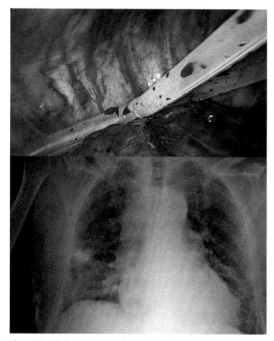

Fig. 12. Right uniportal nonintubated video-assisted wedge resection view. The T-tube intraoperative photograph (*top*) and chest radiograph postoperative control (*bottom*).

Longer bites allow less firing and are money-saving. Conversely, shorter bites are easier to move inside the chest and permit better accomplishment of a curvilinear pathway with an adequate free margin. This may important when removing larger lesions surrounded by bulky parenchyma. The authors prefer the latter devices. Another important trick is the simultaneous use of 2 stapling devices, thus reducing the time between each firing and avoiding the natural reexpansion that occurs after the bite release.

Unless there is a pathology facility in the operating room, the use of frozen sections is not recommended during nonintubated procedures because this step could overly prolong the operating time. This implies accurate patient selection and scheduling only those in whom limited resection is considered the maximal allowed procedure. An adequate free margin should be intraoperatively appreciated and macroscopically assessed on the specimen. For this reason, it is recommended to open the excised parenchyma, thus evaluating the presence and appearance of the resected lesion.

Conversion to Intubation

The need to shift to tracheal intubation during nonintubated VATS originates from either anesthesiologic or surgical reasons. Anesthesiologic reasons of intubation are not the object of this article but can be generically listed as severe hypoxia, persistent hypercapnia, acidosis, inadequate airway patency, hemodynamic instability, insufficient regional pain control, and patient anxiety due to excessive duration of the procedure.[18] The primary surgical reason to consider is difficulty in finding the lesion, which is the main task of the procedure. This could be due to ample and violent lung excursions, scarce pulmonary collapse, thick pleuropulmonary adhesions, or the challenging position of the targeted nodule. Secondarily, intubation may become necessary for massive and persistent hemorrhage during stapling or for the emergent need of unexpected anatomic resection.

Conversion to intubation and general anesthesia can be obtained in lateral decubitus or by turning the patient supine. If turning the patient supine is chosen, 1 thick silk stitch or surgical drapes can momentarily and rapidly keep a small VATS access sterile. The anesthesiologist should ensure the stability of patient's head and neck, and should lead the team to turn the patient back to supine.[10]

DIAGNOSTIC RESECTION

The increasing importance of assessing the biologic identity of the tumor parallels the need to collect the largest possible amount of tissue. Accordingly, even histologically accurate CT-guided needle biopsies may sometimes be inadequate to provide enough quantity of cells for the whole panel of required studies.[19] For this reason, the possibility of resecting the entire nodule with a greater safety using just a slightly more profound anesthesia compared with transcutaneous procedures makes nonintubated procedures very attractive. Another important consideration in favor of a nonintubated VATS biopsy is the safety of the procedure, which has a significantly lower complication rate than CT-guided biopsy, especially in frail patients.[20]

POSTOPERATIVE CARE

Postoperatively, patients are able to resume oral intake, thus fluid intravenous administration can be rapidly suspended. We encourage early ambulation on the same day of surgery.[4] We usually control pain with a moderate opioid-based intravenous analgesia and/or oral multimodal analgesia, according to the needs of the patient.[8,10] In order to remove the chest drain as soon as possible, a sitting chest radiograph is taken between 2 to 8 hours postoperatively. Requirements for chest drain removal are absence of air leak and pleural collection of less than 200 mL in 24 hours.[15] In the case of an air leak lasting more than 6 days, we always try to shift from water seal to Heimlich valve to avoid prolonged aspiration. We find suction portable devices useful, especially those capable of quantifying air leakage. Patients are usually discharged within 3 days after surgery.

COMMENT

Only few years ago, the discovery of lung cancer was related to the onset of late symptoms due to tumor overgrowth. This invariably implied an inoperable neoplasm and these patients were addressed with palliation and symptomatic therapy. Just a few and somewhat lucky cases were incidentally discovered at early stage and benefited from an aggressive surgical treatment.

The increasing diffusion of screening programs, as well as the refinement of diagnostic devices, has recently revolutionized this scenario. Currently, a growing number of small size, multiform, and peripheral lung cancers are increasingly discovered, thus allowing earlier and potentially more radical procedures with less loss of parenchyma.

This kind of surgery requires particular skill in detection and rapidity of execution, and this may be a significant technical limitation. Furthermore,

atypical resection without systemic lymph nodal dissection is not considered the standard surgical procedure for patients with clinical stage I non-small cell lung cancer.[21] However, atypical resection features a lower complication rate, short hospitalization duration, and a high preservation of lung function.[22,23] In some recent studies, sublobar resection has shown equivalent oncological results and survival outcome compared with lobectomy.[24–26] In cases of incomplete fissure or in elderly patients with high comorbidity, limited resection of a peripheral nodule in nonintubated anesthesia must be considered an absolute value.[2]

The lower impact of nonintubated surgery on immunologic competence compared with the effect after general anesthesia has been investigated.[27] This may be crucial in oncological patients. Specifically, nonintubated surgery affects the decrease in postoperative total lymphocyte count and, in particular, natural killer subset.[28] Similtaneously, there is a lower increment of inflammatory markers, such as interleukin-6, interleukin-8, C-reactive protein, procalcitonin, and fibrinogen. All these factors, together with the faster mobilization of the patient, could explain the reduced rate of major complications and 30-day mortality experienced with nonintubated surgery.[28] Conversely, a statically significant advantage of nonintubated procedure on long-term survival has not been demonstrated, whereas a slight advantage can be observed.

Definitely, a real advantage can be appreciated in the reduction of costs owing to shorter global operating time and faster recovery.

In conclusion, the authors affirm that nonintubated VATS resection of peripheral lung cancer is a reliable alternative to more aggressive procedures, especially in elderly and frail patients. Appropriate selection is mandatory for the good results of the procedure.

REFERENCES

1. National Lung Screening Trial Research Team, Aberle DR, Adams AM, Berg CD, et al. Reduced lung-cancer mortality with low-dose computed tomographic screening. N Engl J Med 2011;365: 395–409.
2. Katlic MR, Facktor MA. Non-intubated video-assisted thoracic surgery in patients aged 80 years and older. Ann Transl Med 2015;3:101.
3. Mineo TC. Epidural anesthesia in awake thoracic surgery. Eur J Cardiothorac Surg 2007;32:13–9.
4. Pompeo E, Mineo D, Rogliani P, et al. Feasibility and results of awake thoracoscopic resection of solitary

pulmonary nodules. Ann Thorac Surg 2004;78: 1761–8.

5. Mineo TC, Tacconi F. Monitored anesthesia care thoracic surgery. Thorac Cancer 2014;5:1–13.

6. Gonzalez-Rivas D, Bonome C, Fieira E, et al. Non-intubated video-assisted thoracoscopic lung resections: the future of thoracic surgery? Eur J Cardiothorac Surg 2016;49:721–31.

7. Mineo TC, Tamburini A, Perroni G, et al. 1000 cases of tubeless video-assisted thoracic surgery at the Rome. Future Oncol 2016;12:13–8.

8. Irons JF, Martinez G. Anaesthetic considerations for non-intubated thoracic surgery. J Vis Surg 2016;2:61.

9. Mineo TC, Ambrogi V, Sellitri F. Non-intubated video-assisted surgery from multi to uniportal approaches: single-centre experience. EMJ Respir 2016;4: 104–12.

10. Kiss G, Castillo M. Nonintubated anesthesia in thoracic surgery: general issues. Ann Transl Med 2015;3:110.

11. Rocco G, Martin-Ucar A, Passera E. Uniportal VATS wedge pulmonary resections. Ann Thorac Surg 2004;77:726–8.

12. Mineo TC, Ambrogi V. Surgical techniques for myasthenia gravis: Video-Assisted Thoracic Surgery. Thorac Surg Clin 2019;29:165–75.

13. Rocco G, Martucci N, La Manna C, et al. Ten-year experience on 644 patients undergoing single-port (uniportal) video-assisted thoracoscopic surgery. Ann Thorac Surg 2013;96:434–8.

14. Hung MH, Liu YJ, Hsu HH, et al. Nonintubated video-assisted thoracoscopic surgery for management of indeterminate pulmonary nodules. Ann Transl Med 2015;3:105.

15. Tsai TM, Lin MW, Hsu HH, et al. Nonintubated uniportal thoracoscopic wedge resection for early lung cancer. J Vis Surg 2017;3:155.

16. Gonzalez-Rivas D, Fernandez R, De la Torre M, et al. Single-port thoracoscopic lobectomy in a nonintubated patient: the least invasive procedure for major lung resection? Interact Cardiovasc Thorac Surg 2014;19:552–5.

17. Keating J, Singhal S. Novel methods of intraoperative localization and margin assessment of pulmonary nodules. Semin Thorac Surg 2016;28:127–36.

18. Gonzalez-Rivas D, Aymerich H, Bonome C, et al. Open operations to nonintubated uniportal video-assisted thoracoscopic lobectomy: minimizing the trauma to the patient. Ann Thorac Surg 2015;100: 2003–5.

19. Ilie M, Long-Mira E, Bence C. Comparative study of the PD-L1 status between surgically resected specimens and matched biopsies of NSCLC patients reveal major discordances: a potential issue for anti-PD-L1 therapeutic strategies. Ann Oncol 2016; 27:147–53.

20. Wiener RS, Schwartz LM, Woloshin S, et al. Population-based risk of complications following transthoracic needle lung biopsy of a pulmonary nodule. Ann Intern Med 2011;155:137–44.

21. Howington JA, Blum MG, Chang AC, et al. Treatment of stage I and II non-small cell lung cancer: diagnosis and management of lung cancer, 3rd ed: American College of Chest Physicians evidence-based clinical practice guidelines. Chest 2013;143: e278S–313S.

22. Landreneau RJ, Sugarbaker DJ, Mack MJ, et al. Wedge resection versus lobectomy for stage I (T1 N0 M0) non-small-cell lung cancer. J Thorac Cardiovasc Surg 1997;113:691–700.

23. Keenan RJ, Landreneau RJ, Maley RH Jr, et al. Segmental resection spares pulmonary function in patients with stage I lung cancer. Ann Thorac Surg 2004;78:228–33.

24. Kates M, Swanson S, Wisnivesky JP. Survival following lobectomy and limited resection for the treatment of stage I non-small cell lung cancer≤1 cm in size: a review of SEER data. Chest 2011; 139:491–6.

25. Altorki NK, Yip R, Hanaoka T, et al. Sublobar resection is equivalent to lobectomy for clinical stage 1A lung cancer in solid nodules. J Thorac Cardiovasc Surg 2014;147:754–62.

26. Yano M, Yoshida J, Koike T, et al. Survival of 1737 lobectomy-tolerable patients who underwent limited resection for cStage IA non-small-cell lung cancer. Eur J Cardiothorac Surg 2015;47:135–42.

27. Vanni G, Tacconi F, Sellitri F, et al. Impact of awake videothoracoscopic surgery on postoperative lymphocyte responses. Ann Thorac Surg 2010;90: 973–8.

28. Mineo TC, Sellitri F, Vanni G, et al. Immunological and inflammatory impact of non-intubated lung metastasectomy. Int J Mol Sci 2017;18:1466.

Anatomic Segmentectomy in Nonintubated Video-Assisted Thoracoscopic Surgery

Carlos Gálvez, MD, PhD[a],*, Sergio Bolufer, MD, PhD[a], Elisa Gálvez, MD, PhD[b],
Jose Navarro-Martínez, MD, EDAIC[c], Maria Galiana-Ivars, MD[c],
Julio Sesma, MD[a], María Jesús Rivera-Cogollos, MD[c]

KEYWORDS

- Nonintubated thoracic surgery • Thoracic surgery • Video assisted
- Pulmonary surgical procedures • Sublobar pulmonary resections

KEY POINTS

- Anatomic segmentectomies have become more frequent in the treatment not only of benign lesions and central metastasis but also in early-stage primary lung cancers.
- Nonintubated anatomic segmentectomies can be safely performed under deep sedation with vagal blockade in strictly selected patients.
- Improved postoperative recovery in terms of earlier resumption of oral intake, decreased chest tube duration, and hospital stay has been described.
- Nonintubated anatomic segmentectomy has an incidence of complications comparable with conventional intubation, and does not affect the quality of lymph node dissection in lung cancer.

 Video content accompanies this article at http://www.thoracic.theclinics.com.

INTRODUCTION

Nonintubated anatomic resections under spontaneous breathing have spread widely within the last years, although they are not routinely performed in many thoracic surgery units. There are still many concerns about indications, technical details, and potential advantages and risks that should be first addressed.[1]

The main challenges while facing major resections under spontaneous breathing are the need for a stable mediastinum, the control of cough reflex by vagal block, the balance of sedation, and the duration of the surgery to avoid respiratory depression and severe hypercapnia.

Anatomic segmentectomy has been considered for many years an alternative only for high-risk patients deemed inoperable for lobar resection because of decreased pulmonary function, because the idea of higher risk of recurrence has been well established since 1995.[2] However, as minimally invasive thoracic surgery developed, the idea of lung-sparing resection became more interesting. Were all the cases of non–small cell lung cancer or other central lesions candidates for lobar resection, or could surgeons spare lung parenchyma in specific cases? Many studies proved that sublobar resections, especially anatomic segmentectomies, were oncologically optimal for some cases of early-stage lung

Conflict of interest: The authors have no conflicts of interest.
[a] Thoracic Surgery Department, Hospital General Universitario Alicante, C/Pintor Baeza, 12, Alicante 03010, Spain; [b] Medical Oncology, Hospital General Universitario Elda, Ctra. Sax- La Torreta, S/N, Elda, Alicante 03600, Spain; [c] Anesthesiology and Surgical Critical Care Department, Hospital General Universitario Alicante, C/Pintor Baeza, 12, Alicante 03010, Spain
* Corresponding author.
E-mail address: carlos.galvez.cto@gmail.com

cancer,[3-6] and, as the knowledge and techniques evolved, these resections were extended to central benign lesions and metastases, as well as multicenter preinvasive or minimally invasive lesions or second primary tumors.

The combination of minimally invasive approach in terms of video-assisted techniques (video-assisted thoracoscopic surgery [VATS]), lung-sparing resections, and less aggressive anesthesia methods promises to be an attractive new approach in thoracic surgery: less invasive and more physiologic.

ANATOMIC SEGMENTECTOMY

Sublobar anatomic resections include lung resections of segments and subsegments with division of both vascular and bronchial structures, and thus include anatomic segmentectomy. These procedures have especially spread within the last decade because of the diffusion and development of minimally invasive thoracic surgery, and the concept of lung-sparing surgery, which means safely preserving as much lung parenchyma as possible.[6-12] A comprehensive knowledge is required of pulmonary anatomy in terms of intralobar segmental and subsegmental divisions, and the most frequent anatomic variations in arterial, venous, and bronchial division. There are not many reports that specifically analyze the anatomic patterns.[10,11]

The main expected benefit is the preservation of more lung parenchyma, thus the absolute loss of postoperative lung function is lower than for lobar and supralobar resections. Most published studies have not addressed the functional repercussion, but an article by Charloux and Quoix[13] in 2017 reported a lower decrease in postoperative forced expiratory volume in the first second (FEV1) at 12 months compared with lobectomy (5% vs 11%), a lower decrease in global pulmonary function in patients with diminished preoperative lung function, and a direct relation between the number of resected segments and the functional loss. Curiously, there are no studies that specifically address the reduction of lung function in relation to the surgical approach (VATS, open thoracotomy), and the loss of function within the early postoperative (first days or weeks) compared with lobar resections.

Anatomic segmentectomy has been used in the treatment of several disorders, mainly benign lesions centrally located in the lobe, pulmonary metastasis, and early-stage lung cancer.[14] Since the Lung Cancer Study Group report in 1995, sublobar resections (anatomic and wedge) have shown a higher recurrence and death rate in tumors less than 3 cm in diameter, so lobectomy was set as the standard surgical treatment of early-stage lung cancer.[2] Since then, there have been published many studies that prove that anatomic sublobar resections show the same disease-free and overall survival as lobectomy for tumors less than 2 cm,[4,6,7,15-17] so sublobar anatomic resections have been included in the main clinical guidelines as an accepted procedure for early-stage adenocarcinoma less than 2 cm, in peripheral locations without nodal involvement.[18,19]

The available evidence points to equivalent outcomes in terms of survival, a lower rate of postoperative , and a better postoperative profile (chest tube duration, hospital stay). Nevertheless, it is necessary to highlight that most published studies are case series or comparative unicentric studies but there is still a lack of multicenter studies and randomized trials.

NONINTUBATED VIDEO-ASSISTED THORACOSCOPIC SURGERY
Benefits of Nonintubated Video-assisted Thoracoscopic Surgery

Despite the lack of comparative studies, thoracic surgery in awake patients has shown a decrease in overall postoperative stay and duration of chest tube compared with the traditional intubated approach.[20-25] Likewise, a lower rate of postoperative complications has been reported in certain procedures,[21,23] and a cost reduction.[22] Most noncomparative studies, such as case series or isolated case reports, show the feasibility of this approach for the management of most procedures in thoracic surgery.[26,27]

As with awake nonintubated surgery, there are few randomized or comparative studies of nonintubated surgery in unawake patients. The results point to a decrease in the rate of postoperative complications, even in the case of anatomic pulmonary resections.[28-30] A shorter anesthesia time, a higher occupational ratio in the operating room, a shorter postanesthetic recovery, and a shorter hospital stay have also been described.[31,32]

Table 1 shows the main outcomes of nonintubated awake and unawake approaches in different types of pulmonary resections.[23-25,28-30,33-35]

Technical Aspects of Nonintubated Video-assisted Thoracoscopic Surgery

Sedation/general anesthesia
Anatomic segmentectomy under nonintubated VATS (unawake) requires deep sedation (Ramsay Sedation Scale >3)[36] or even general anesthesia.

Table 1
Main benefits of nonintubated approach for different pulmonary resections

Procedure	Study	Author, Year	Main Benefits
Primary spontaneous pneumothorax	RCT	Pompeo et al,[25] 2007	Fewer side effects (vomiting, urinary retention)
Secondary spontaneous pneumothorax	PSM	Noda et al,[28] 2012	Lower postoperative respiratory complication rate
Lung volume reduction surgery	RCT	Pompeo et al,[23] 2012	Lower overall morbidity
Pulmonary metastasis	NRC	Pompeo et al,[24] 2007	Lower hospital stay
Minor VATS procedures	NRC	Irons et al,[33] 2017	Shorter anesthesia time, less postoperative moderate-severe pain
VATS lobectomies	NRC	Chen et al,[29] 2011	Less postoperative morbidity (lower complication rate)
Lung cancer in the elderly	NRC	Wu et al,[35] 2013	Lower postoperative delirium rate
Multiple indications	RCT	Liu et al,[30] 2015	Less postoperative morbidity (lower respiratory complication rate)
Pulmonary anatomic resections (segmentectomy and lobectomy)	PSM	Liu et al,[34] 2016	Earlier resumption of oral intake, less pleural fluid drainage, and shorter hospital stay

Abbreviations: NRC, nonrandomized comparative; PSM, propensity score matching analysis; RCT, randomized controlled trial.

By administering intravenous agents such as propofol (target-controlled infusion), the patient is maintained with a Bispectral Index (BIS) between 40 and 60,[37,38] although experienced groups recommend an even deeper anesthesia (BIS 30–50). By administering other agents, such as fentanyl,[38] remifentanyl,[39] sufentanil, or dexmedetomidine,[40] the depth of sedation/anesthesia is kept constant. The main risk from deeper sedation is hypercapnia, which, if it exceeds the permissive limits ($Paco_2 > 55$ mm Hg), can increase the frequency and depth of breathing and the mediastinal balance, making the procedure difficult, as well as the risk of respiratory acidosis.

Locoregional analgesia

There are several ways to perform analgesia, with epidural analgesia, paravertebral block, and selective intercostal block being the most reported. Although it is not the subject of this article, some key concepts are highlighted.

- Epidural analgesia has been the gold standard for regional analgesia in nonintubated VATS. A somatosensory and motor block is performed, usually using drugs such as ropivacaine at different concentrations,[41] or in combination with sufentanyl,[42] with lidocaine and sufentanyl.[43] Bupivacaine has also been used at different concentrations.[44]

- Paravertebral blockade. As an alternative to epidural anesthesia, a paravertebral block/catheter may be performed. The paravertebral block is unilateral, produces no sympathetic block, and has a lower rate of respiratory complications, urinary retention, and hypotension.[45] The use of ropivacaine has been described at different concentrations.

- Intercostal blockade. Selective intercostal block can be performed under direct view of the desired intercostal nerves with bupivacaine,[38] and also percutaneously injected ropivacaine has been reported.[45] The authors routinely perform intercostal blocks from the third to seventh intercostal posterior spaces,[46] with bupivacaine 0.5%, 1 to 1.5 mL in each space at the beginning of the procedure, and at the end of the procedure; before closing the incision, we repeat the block, and sometimes extend it to the second intercostal space for relieving the pain occasioned by the tip of the chest tube (Video 1).

Intercostal block is a more selective unilateral block, without systemic adverse events (urinary retention, constipation).

Oxygenation/respiratory support

Nonintubated VATS can be performed without the need for additional oxygenation,[47] but oxygen supplementation through Venturi facial masks is commonly reported.[41,48] In addition, the use of conventional nasal prongs, high-flow oxygen delivery nasal prongs,[41] and nasopharyngeal cannulas[49] has also been described, in order to avoid hypoxemia during the procedure. These devices increase the fraction of oxygen in the inspired air to optimize oxygenation. Supraglottic devices such as the laryngeal mask have also been described.[31,39,50] The aim is to keep a breathing rate of between 12 and 20 breaths per minute, to avoid tachypnea, which can lead to deeper breathing and an oscillating surgical field. With these devices, good tissue oxygenation is achieved and hypoxemia is avoided. The laryngeal mask allows for easier conversion to tracheal intubation in the event of an intraoperative complication.[31] **Fig. 1** summarizes some of the most frequently used devices for oxygenation.

Oxygenation can be ensured through these techniques, but the main concerns focus on the risk of hypercapnia. Secondary to rebreathing and deep sedation needed for anatomic resections, moderate hypercapnia is usually observed. In cases of severe hypercapnia, the authors reduce the propofol infusion and we assist the patient with the facial mask until recovering normal parameters, but, if severe hypercapnia remains, conversion to tracheal intubation and mechanical ventilation should be considered, especially in patients with some degree of pulmonary compromise.

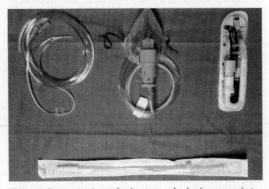

Fig. 1. Oxygenation devices used during nonintubated procedures: from left to right on the top, nasal prongs, facial mask, high-flow oxygen nasal prongs. At the bottom, nasopharyngeal cannula.

Cough reflex: vagal block

Cough reflex during a nonintubated procedure can make it challenging to perform or even lead to a complication, so several methods have been used for its control (atropine in premedication, intravenous or aerosolized lidocaine), the most effective being direct vagal block with bupivacaine 0.5%, 2 to 3 mL in the low right paratracheal region or aortopulmonary window in procedures in the right and left hemithorax respectively[51] (Video 2). Left vagal block is best performed by pulling the lung gently anteriorly and incising the mediastinal pleura just after the laryngeal recurrent nerve visualization. Vagal block ensures cough abolition for 12 hours so most anatomic resections can be safely performed. It is better to block the vagal transmission before initiating parenchyma or bronchial pulling maneuvers in order to avoid cough reflex triggering. It is mandatory for safely performing anatomic resections such as anatomic segmentectomies.

ANATOMIC SEGMENTECTOMY IN NONINTUBATED VIDEO-ASSISTED THORACOSCOPIC SURGERY
Starting Point

Before embarking on a nonintubated program for anatomic segmentectomies, a learning curve for operating minor procedures is mandatory, in order to develop skills for all the members of the multidisciplinary team, and to achieve a comprehensive knowledge of the physiology of surgical pneumothorax in spontaneously breathing patients. Pulmonary biopsies, metastatectomies, and pneumothorax should first be attempted to find out the main difficulties and the possible solutions.[52,53] Patients with primary spontaneous pneumothorax are usually young and healthy patients with preserved cough reflex, so surgeons can safely manage the first attempts of vagal block and test the outcomes.

The VATS experience of the surgeon is relevant because nonintubated VATS anatomic segmentectomy defies the surgical capability to operate on a less stable mediastinal/surgical field. It is advisable to begin nonintubated major resections with highly experienced surgeons in VATS, able to manage intraoperative complications (ie, major bleedings) and complex procedures such as sleeve lobectomies in order to achieve abilities such as primary sutures for a potential bleed.[54]

It is also recommended that anesthesiologists first develop a lateral decubitus orotracheal intubation learning curve and simulations of emergent intubation in an experimental model.[55] The nursing team should be familiar with the essential details of the whole procedure and the management of critical potential situations. They must know their exact roles in the different steps of the procedure, and it is important to make them part of the successful development of these complex resections. The objective of these programs should focus on decreasing global invasiveness of the surgical procedure, preserving the safety, decreasing postoperative complications, and improving the antitumor immune profile.

Indications

Strictly selecting patients for nonintubated anatomic segmentectomy is extremely important, because these procedures combine both challenging surgical aspects with a complex environment, as described earlier.

Selection should be done in 2 steps: first, selecting cases for anatomic segmentectomy (**Box 1**); second, selecting patients for nonintubated VATS.

Anatomic segmentectomy can be performed in benign lesions centrally located in the lung (ie, benign pneumocytomas), carcinoid tumors, and pulmonary metastasis not amenable to wedge resections with safe margins.

Anatomic segmentectomy has shown comparable oncological outcomes in terms of recurrence-free and overall survival in early-stage lung cancer. What still needs to be clarified is which early-stage lung cancers can safely be subjected to anatomic segmentectomy. The latest version of the main clinical guidelines supports anatomic segmentectomy in lung cancer for specific circumstances. The European Society of Medical Oncology (ESMO) guidelines propose sublobar resection for less than or equal to 2-cm pure ground-glass opacity (GGO) lesions, or adenocarcinoma in situ (AIS), or minimally invasive adenocarcinoma (MIA), but state that lobectomy should be preferred for solid lesions less than 2 cm in diameter.[19] The National Comprehensive Cancer Network (NCCN) states for non–small cell lung cancer that segmentectomy (preferred) or wedge resection is appropriate in selected patients for the following reasons[18]:

- Poor pulmonary reserve or other major comorbidity that contraindicates lobectomy
- Peripheral nodule less than or equal to 2 cm with at least 1 of the following:
  o Pure AIS histology
  o Nodule has greater than or equal to 50% ground-glass appearance on computed tomography (CT)
  o Radiologic surveillance confirms a long doubling time (≥400 days)

> **Box 1**
> **Indications for anatomic segmentectomy**
>
> Centrally located benign lesions
>
> Carcinoid tumors
>
> Pulmonary metastasis not amenable for wedge resection
>
> Primary lung cancer
>
> - Second primary lung cancer with past history of pulmonary resection
> - Multiple multilobe pure GGO lesions (atypical adenomatous hyperplasia, AIS, MIA, lepidic predominant adenocarcinoma)
> - Poor pulmonary reserve or other major comorbidity that contraindicates lobectomy
> - Peripheral nodule less than or equal to 2 cm with at least 1 of the following:
>   o Pure AIS histology
>   o Nodule has greater than or equal to 50% ground-glass appearance on computed tomography
>   o Radiologic surveillance confirms a long doubling time (≥400 days)
> - Peripheral tumors less than or equal to 2 cm in maximum diameter, without nodal involvement neither metastasis, regardless of histologic subtype and radiological appearance, with intraoperative lymph node assessment including intralobar N1 stations, and free resection margins of at least 1 cm or tumor diameter size
>
> *Abbreviations:* AIS, adenocarcinoma in situ; GGO, ground-glass opacity; MIA, minimally invasive adenocarcinoma.

Multiple multilobe GGO lesions, past history of solid neoplasms without the possibility of differentiation between primary lung cancer and distant metastasis, and second primary tumors in patients previously operated are also indications for anatomic segmentectomy.[3,34]

However, there are many studies that have shown comparable oncological outcomes for anatomic segmentectomy in peripheral tumors less than 2 cm in maximum diameter, without nodal involvement or metastasis, regardless of histologic subtype and radiological appearance.[6,15–17] There is even a 2014 meta-analysis that showed no differences in overall and cancer-specific survival for anatomic segmentectomy compared with lobectomy in stage IA tumors less than 2 cm in diameter.[4] Nowadays surgical groups with experience in anatomic sublobar resections are performing these lung-sparing techniques not only in pure GGO, AIS, or MIA less than 2 cm without nodal or metastatic involvement but also in early-stage adenocarcinomas less than 2 cm without nodal or metastatic involvement (although with solid component), but what most highlight is the need for intraoperative lymph node assessment, including intralobar N1 stations, and free resection margins of at least 1 cm or tumor diameter size.

There are no standardized selection criteria for nonintubated VATS procedures, although several teams have reported their algorithms (**Fig. 2**). Despite the initial reports of the team from Tor Vergata University (Rome, Italy)[21–25] with severely emphysematous patients, most surgical teams that have developed nonintubated anatomic resection programs have globally selected a propitious profile of populations: no obesity, no severe comorbidities, no underlying pulmonary disease, solitary pulmonary nodule including early-stage lung cancer, metastatic or benign disease.[30,56,57]

In our nonintubated program initiated in 2013, we set the inclusion and exclusion criteria for these procedures as described in **Boxes 2** and **3**.[55]

We initially consider patients more than 18 years old without prohibitive pulmonary function tests and low-moderate American Society of Anesthesiologists anesthesia risk score (ASA $\leq$ 3). The main contraindications are obesity, patients with unfavorable anatomy, previous spine surgery or thoracotomy, coagulation disorders or locally advanced lung cancers (cT4), hemodynamically unstable patients, or expected extensive pleural adhesions that prolong surgical time.

These criteria are not absolute and have been developed through achieving experience in nonintubated procedures but must be updated regarding the continuous improvement. They reflect an attempt to include patients for nonintubated uniportal anatomic resections with favorable conditions in terms of anatomy, global health status of the patient, and tumor stage but, depending on the center, selection criteria may differ and there are no standardized criteria. **Fig. 2**. summarizes de indications for both anatomical segmentectomies and nonintubated procedure, as well as the cornerstones for developing this less invasive approach.

Surgical Technique

In general, anatomic segmentectomy under nonintubated VATS can be safely performed in the same manner as in intubated patients, as long as a combination of locoregional analgesia (intercostal blockade, paravertebral, and epidural) and vagal blockade has successfully been performed. Vagal blockade is mandatory because pulling maneuvers and segmental bronchial dissection can trigger the cough reflex, which could be challenging while performing vascular dissection.

Bronchovascular structures should be divided individually, avoiding what the authors call half-segmentectomies, in which several structures are

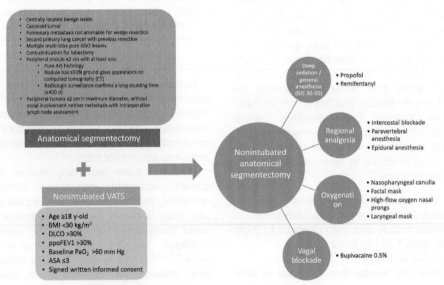

Fig. 2. The selection criteria for anatomic segmentectomy and nonintubated approach and the cornerstones during the procedure. ASA, American Society of Anesthesiologists anesthesia risk score; AIS, adenocarcinoma in situ; BMI, body mass index; DLCO, diffusing capacity for carbon monoxide; ppoFEV1, predicted postoperative forced expiratory volume in the first second.

Box 2
Inclusion criteria for nonintubated video-assisted thoracoscopic surgery anatomic segmentectomy

Age greater than or equal to 18 years

DLCO greater than 30%

Predicted postoperative FEV_1 greater than 30%

Baseline Pao_2 greater than 60 mm Hg

ASA less than or equal to 3

Signed written informed consent

Abbreviations: ASA, American Society of Anesthesiology; DLCO, diffusion capacity of the lung for carbon monoxide; FEV_1, forced expiratory volume in the first second.

Box 3
Exclusion criteria for nonintubated video-assisted thoracoscopic surgery anatomic segmentectomy

1. Unfavorable anatomy
   1.1. BMI greater than 30
   1.2. Narrow thorax
   1.3. Expected difficult airway
       1.3.1. Prominent superior incisors
       1.3.2. Impossibility of occluding the superior lip with the inferior incisors
       1.3.3. Mouth opening less than 3 cm
       1.3.4. Mallampati score greater than 2
       1.3.5. Arcuate or tight palate
       1.3.6. Rigid, indurated, or nonelastic maxillar space
       1.3.7. Thyroid-to-chin distance less than 6 cm
       1.3.8. Short or wide neck
       1.3.9. Abnormal cervical flexoextension
2. Previous surgery in cervical/thoracic spine
3. Previous ipsilateral thoracotomy (not previous VATS)
4. Uncontrolled gastroesophageal regurgitation
5. Hemodynamically unstable patient
6. Pleural adhesions in more than 50% of pleural surface
7. Coagulation disorders
8. Clinical stage cT4 lung cancer
9. Induction radiotherapy

Abbreviation: BMI, body mass index.

---

not individually dissected and divided together en block. In some specific segmentectomies, 1 segmental vein can be divided together with the fissure after previous individual dissection taking care of structures from the remaining segments.

Preoperative tridimensional reconstructions have become more useful,[8] in order to more accurately define the segmental location of the lesion and plan the resection of isolated segments or combined segmentectomies to achieve safe resection margins. However, careful examination of the preoperative conventional CT scan gives useful information, and many procedures can be preoperatively planned without the use of three-dimensional reconstructions.

Before dividing the segmental bronchus, the authors usually clamp it and reventilate to check and define the intersegmental plane. This process can also be done under a nonintubated approach, by means of facial ventilation masks tightly applied to the patient and actively ventilating, in the same manner in which air leaks are checked after nonintubated procedures (Video 3). The intersegmental plane can be safely divided using endostaplers or advanced energy devices.

Results

Randomized trials and comparative studies

There are no randomized trials comparing nonintubated versus intubated VATS anatomic segmentectomies. There is only 1 comparative Chinese study published in 2016 by Guo and colleagues.[9] The study analyzes the short-term outcomes in a 5-year experience of 140 segmentectomies by the 3-port technique, including 48 segmentectomies performed under epidural anesthesia and laryngeal mask, with propofol, dexmedetomidine, and also under vagal block. Mean peak end-tidal

CO_2 of the nonintubated group was higher (44.81 vs 33.15 mm Hg, $P<.001$), whereas nonintubated segmentectomy also had lower white blood count (6.08 $\times$ 109 vs 7.75 $\times$ 109, $P = .004$), lower anesthesia cost (¥5757.19 vs ¥7401.85, $P<.001$), shorter duration of postoperative chest tube drainage (2.25 vs 3.16 days, $P = .047$), earlier resumption of oral intake (6.76 vs 17.58 hours, $P<.001$), and a trend toward shorter postoperative hospital stays (6.04 vs 7.83 days, $P = .057$) than the intubated group. They found comparable results in terms of operative time (2.81 vs 2.74 hours, $P = .643$), intraoperative blood loss (75.10 vs 56.65 mL, $P = .441$), numbers of dissected lymph nodes of patients with primary non–small cell lung cancer (8.06 vs 8.02, $P = .969$), chest tube drainage volume (383.46 vs 626.98 mL, $P = .145$), and intraoperative lowest Spo_2 (oxygen saturation by pulse oximetry; 98.0% vs 96.8%, $P = .422$). There was only 1 conversion to intubated anesthesia in the nonintubated group (2.1%) caused by excessive mediastinal movement, and 1 conversion to thoracotomy in the intubated group caused by uncontrolled bleeding.

The complication incidences in both groups were comparable ($P = .248$). Four complications developed in 4 patients (8.3%) in the nonintubated group (pneumonia, chylothorax, and pulmonary embolism), and 14 complications developed in 14 patients (15.2%) in the intubated group (including pneumonia, chylothorax, bleeding requiring thoracotomy, pulmonary atelectasis, sputum retention requiring bronchoscopy, brain infarction, deep venous thrombosis, subcutaneous emphysema, and cardiac arrhythmia). There was no mortality in either group. The investigators concluded that nonintubated anatomic segmentectomy is feasible and safe compared with traditional intubated anesthesia, highlighting a shorter postoperative recovery in terms of chest tube duration, hospital stay, and resumption of oral intake, without increasing the complication incidence.

The same group also published in 2016 a propensity score matching analysis of early outcomes on video-assisted thoracic surgery for non–small cell lung cancer regarding the type of anesthesia.[34] They selected 363 cases of lobectomy or anatomic segmentectomy within a 3-year period. They excluded 24 patients, so 151 patients were eventually operated under nonintubated VATS, including 32 anatomic segmentectomies. They performed a propensity score matching, so the analysis included 20 nonintubated and 20 intubated anatomic segmentectomies. After this matching in the segmentectomy groups, the nonintubated group showed significant differences from the intubated group regarding postoperative fasting time (6.5 ± 2.1 vs 13.8 ± 2.3 hours), mean volume of postoperative pleural fluid drainage (354.5 vs 723.0 mL), and mean duration of postoperative hospital stay (6.0 vs 8.3 days, $P<.05$). No significant differences occurred between the two groups in terms of intraoperative blood loss (49.5 ± 10.1 vs 57.0 ± 76.2 mL), surgical duration (152.5 ± 34.8 vs 158.3 ± 48.8 min), postoperative complications (15% vs 15%) or lymph nodes sampled (numbers, 7.8 ± 5.4 vs 6.4 ± 5.3; stations, 3.2 ± 1.4 vs 2.7 ± 1.5), and a trend toward reduction of chest tube duration (2.6 ± 1.2 vs 4.3 ± 7.2 days, $P = .310$).

The investigators concluded that nonintubated anatomic segmentectomy was safe and showed a better postoperative profile with a decrease in postoperative pleural fluid drainage, hospital stay, and resumption of oral intake, which were the same benefits observed in the lobectomy nonintubated group compared with the intubated control group. The investigators hypothesized that nonintubated surgery may affect the autonomic response less, preserving better gastrointestinal motility decreasing postoperative fasting time, which as a result could improve metabolism and absorption of nutrients, decreasing pleural exudation. The number of lymph nodes dissected in both groups during segmentectomy showed no significant differences (7.8 ± 5.4 vs 6.4 ± 5.3, $P = .412$, in the nonintubated and intubated groups respectively). Nevertheless, the study has 2 important limitations: first, the investigators excluded from the analysis all the conversions from nonintubated to intubated anesthesia, thus avoiding an intention-to-treat analysis, despite all conversions being in the lobectomy group; second, in the segmentectomy groups, they performed only lymph node sampling instead of systematic lymph node dissection, so the complication rate could be affected by this less exhaustive lymph node assessment.

Noncomparative studies

Most published studies are descriptive series, some large case series, describing their results with nonintubated anatomic segmentectomies.

In 2012, Chen and colleagues[56] reported their 3-year experience with 285 cases using a 3-port VATS technique. Procedures were performed under moderate sedation (Ramsay score III),[36] epidural analgesia, and with ventilation mask and vagal blockade. They included 16 anatomic segmentectomies, thus representing 5.6% of the total sample. There was only 1 conversion to tracheal intubation in the segmentectomy group, representing a 6.3% conversion rate. The total complication rate of the study was 3.9%, including prolonged air leak, bleeding, and pneumonia, and there was no mortality or major complications. Hypercapnia was noted, especially in long procedures, but was always permissive and did not affect hemodynamics. Vagal block led to cough reflex abolishment without affecting heart rate, breathing rate, or blood pressure, and is essential to perform in anatomic resections in which bronchial dissection is mandatory, potentially triggering a cough reflex.[57] The investigators highlighted that, with their described nonintubated technique, both diagnostic and therapeutic procedures can be performed safely.

The same group presented in 2013 their initial experience with nonintubated anatomic segmentectomy for lung tumors[58] with the technique previously described. Twenty-one segmentectomies were included, with a median tumor size of 1.5 cm, and an FEV1 of 105.5%. Of these, 76.2% were malignant tumors, with 13 cases of non–small cell lung cancer (4 compromised and 9 intentional segmentectomies). Most segmentectomies were conventional (80.9%), including left apical trisegmentectomy, lingulectomy, and lower lobe upper segmentectomies. Mean highest Pa_{CO_2} was 51.8 mm Hg, and there was only 1 conversion to tracheal intubation (4.8%), caused by vigorous mediastinal and diaphragm movement in a patient with body mass index (BMI) more than 30 kg/m^2. Only 1 patient experienced postoperative complication in terms of air leak lasting more than 3 days (4.8%). Mean chest tube duration was 2.5 days and mean hospital stay 6 days. The study was mainly limited by its retrospective design and small sample size.

In 2014 the same group described their first report of nonintubated uniportal segmentectomy, describing their changes to the anesthetic management: they started to perform target control infusion sedation with propofol along with intrathoracic intercostal and vagal blockade.[12]

A study from another group in 2014, by Guo and colleagues,[59] reported their initial 2-year experience of complete thoracoscopic nonintubated anatomic segmentectomies. The procedures were performed with a multiport VATS technique, under epidural analgesia, remifentanil and propofol infusion, nasopharyngeal mask ventilation, and vagal blockade. Of these cases, 73.4% were malignancies, with 66.7% of the total sample addressing primary lung adenocarcinoma. There were more different anatomic segmentectomies than in the previous series. There were no perioperative deaths, 1 intraoperative bleeding controlled thoracoscopically, and 2 postoperative complications in the form of postoperative bleeding (13.4%), without any conversion to tracheal intubation. Mean chest tube duration was 2 days, and mean hospital stay 5 days. The investigators emphasized that, 4 to 6 hours after the surgery, patients could resume oral intake and get out of bed. The biggest challenge that the investigators observed was the mediastinal movement, which they put attributed to a higher intrapleural pressure in the nondependent lung compared with the dependent lung, which limits expansion of the contralateral lung. To mitigate the impact of the mediastinal swing during surgery, anesthesiologists can increase the amount of opioids based on the operation, and reduce the breathing frequency

or the respiratory tidal volume, thereby reducing the amplitude of the swing.

In 2015, a review article by Liu and colleagues[57] highlighted how the conversion rate to intubated anesthesia during nonintubated VATS significantly decreases as experience is achieved, For the following reasons: (1) anesthesiologists progressively improve their capabilities in dealing with various complicated conditions such as hypoxemia and hypercapnia during procedures; (2) with accumulated experience, the surgeons are more self-confident and do not easily switch the anesthetic mode when facing amenable problems such as extensive pleural adhesions, small tumors (<6 cm in diameter), and invasion of bronchus, which used to be the contraindications of VATS; (3) the surgical maneuvers become smoother, so difficult actions such as lifting and compression are avoided and, by doing so, the operation has less stimulation on the lung hilum and thus reduces the swinging of mediastinum; and (4) the medical team adapts to the surgical operation under spontaneous breathing, making the whole operation process much smoother.

In 2016 Mineo and colleagues[60] published their 1000-case experience with nonintubated procedures, and reported 36 lung cancer segmentectomies, without specific data about intraoperative and postoperative results.

In 2017, our group published the second report of nonintubated uniportal VATS anatomic segmentectomy (left lower lobe upper segment) after chemotherapy in a pulmonary metastasis.[46] The patient resumed oral intake 6 hours after the surgery, and began walking at postoperative day 1. There was no air leak so the chest tube was removed at 24 hours, and the patient was discharged home on the second postoperative day without complications (Video 4).

SUMMARY

Thoracic surgery has mostly evolved into a minimally invasive surgery, in terms of not only surgical approach but also less aggressive anesthesia protocols and lung-sparing pulmonary resections. This combination has proved attractive for surgeons who want more physiologic thoracic surgery. Indications for anatomic segmentectomies are slowly growing, but it seems that the full potential has not been reached yet.

Nonintubated anatomic resections have developed mainly in unawake protocols with 4 cornerstones: deep sedation, regional analgesia techniques, oxygenation support, and vagal blockade. Without this, the scenario turns into more of a challenge than a practice that could potentially be generalized. Strict selection criteria by excluding difficult cases, obese patients, and patients with severe comorbidities are basic starting points, and previous experience with nonintubated minor procedures in a multidisciplinary team is essential.

Previous studies show significantly shorter postoperative recovery in terms of chest tube duration, hospital stay, and resumption of oral intake, without increasing the complication incidence, and with conversion rates within the expected limits. Despite this, there is a need for standardizing nonintubated anatomic resections and developing prospective multicenter randomized trials to assess the safety and potential advantages. In the authors' opinion, an international nonintubated anatomic resection-working group should be set up in order to strictly collect and analyze data, so individual working groups in nonintubated anatomic resections should combine their efforts.

ACKNOWLEDGMENTS

The authors would like to honor the memory of Prof. Tommaso Claudio Mineo, who unexpectedly passed away recently while we were working on this special issue he enthusiastically led. His contribution to the knowledge in nonintubated surgery is well known worldwide, but we would like to highlight that only people who hesitate about conventional practice and search for alternative pathways push science and innovation forward. May Prof. Mineo rest in peace.

SUPPLEMENTARY DATA

Supplementary data related to this article can be found online at https://doi.org/10.1016/j.thorsurg.2019.09.003.

REFERENCES

1. Mineo TC, Tacconi F. Nonintubated thoracic surgery: a lead role or just a walk on part? Chin J Cancer Res 2014;26:507–10.
2. Ginsberg RJ, Rubinstein LV. Randomized trial of lobectomy versus limited resection for T1 N0 non-small cell lung cancer. Ann Thorac Surg 1995;60:615–22.
3. Martin-Ucar AE, Roel MD. Indication for VATS sublobar resections in early lung cancer. J Thorac Dis 2013;5(SUPPL.3):S194–9.
4. Bao F, Ye P, Yang Y, et al. Segmentectomy or lobectomy for early stage lung cancer: a meta-analysis. Eur J Cardiothorac Surg 2014;46:1–7.
5. Liu Y, Huang C, Liu H, et al. Sublobectomy versus lobectomy for stage IA (T1a) non-small-cell lung cancer: a meta-analysis study. World J Surg Oncol 2014;12:138.
6. D Dziedzic R, Zurek W, Marjański T, et al. Stage I non-small-cell lung cancer: Long-term results of lobectomy versus sublobar resection from the Polish National Lung Cancer Registry. Eur J Cardiothorac Surg 2017;52:363–9.
7. Altorki NK, Kamel MK, Narula N, et al. Anatomical segmentectomy and wedge resections are associated with comparable outcomes for patients with small cT1N0 non-small cell lung cancer. J Thorac Oncol 2016;11:1984–92.
8. Gossot D, Lutz J, Grigoroiu M, et al. Thoracoscopic anatomic segmentectomies for lung cancer: technical aspects. J Vis Surg 2016;2:171.
9. Guo Z, Yin W, Pan H, et al. Video-assisted thoracoscopic surgery segmentectomy by non- intubated or intubated anesthesia: a comparative analysis of short-term outcome. J Thorac Dis 2016;8:359–68.
10. Nagashima T, Shimizu K, Ohtaki Y, et al. An analysis of variations in the bronchovascular pattern of the right upper lobe using three-dimensional CT angiography and bronchography. Gen Thorac Cardiovasc Surg 2015;63:354–60.
11. Nagashima T, Shimizu K, Ohtaki Y, et al. Analysis of variation in bronchovascular pattern of the right middle and lower lobes of the lung using three-dimensional CT angiography and bronchography. Gen Thorac Cardiovasc Surg 2017;65:343–9.
12. Hung M, Cheng Y, Hsu H. Nonintubated uniportal thoracoscopic segmentectomy for lung cancer. J Thorac Cardiovasc Surg 2014;148:e234–5.
13. Charloux A, Quoix E. Lung segmentectomy: does it offer a real functional benefit over lobectomy? Eur Respir Rev 2017;26:170079.
14. Traibi A, Grigoroiu M, Boulitrop C, et al. Predictive factors for complications of anatomical pulmonary Segmentectomies. Interact Cardiovasc Thorac Surg 2013;17:838–44.
15. Song CY, Sakai T, Kimura D, et al. Comparison of perioperative and oncological outcomes between video-assisted segmentectomy and lobectomy for patients with clinical stage IA non-small cell lung cancer: a propensity score matching study. J Thorac Dis 2018;10:4891–901.
16. Cao J, Yuan P, Wang Y, et al. Survival rates after lobectomy, segmentectomy, and wedge resection for non-small cell lung cancer. Ann Thorac Surg 2018;105:1483–91.
17. Moon MH, Moon YK, Moon SW. Segmentectomy versus lobectomy in early non-small cell lung cancer of 2 cm or less in size: a population-based study. Respirology 2018;23:695–703.
18. Ettinger DS, Wood DE, Aisner DL. Non-small cell lung cancer. Version 5. 2017, NCCN clinical practice guidelines in Oncology. J Natl Compr Canc Netw 2017;15(4):504–35.

19. Vansteenkiste J, Crino L, Dooms C, et al. 2nd ESMO Consensus Conference on Lung Cancer: early stage non-small cell lung cancer consensus on diagnosis, treatment and follow-up. Ann Oncol 2014;25: 1462–74.

20. Cajozzo M, Lo Iacono G, Raffaele F, et al. Thoracoscopy in pleural effusion–two techniques: awake single-access video-assisted thoracic surgery versus 2-ports videoassisted thoracic surgery under general anesthesia. Future Oncol 2015;11:39–41.

21. Mineo T, Sellitri F, Tacconi F, et al. Quality of life and outcomes after nonintubated versus intubated videothoracoscopic pleurodesis for malignant pleural effusion: comparison by a case-matched study. J Palliat Med 2014;17:761–8.

22. Pompeo E, Dauri M. Is there any benefit in using awake anesthesia with thoracic epidural in thoracoscopic talc pleurodesis? J Thorac Cardiovasc Surg 2013;146:495–7.e1.

23. Pompeo E, Rogliani P, Tacconi F, et al. Randomized comparison of awake nonresectional versus nonawake resectional lung volume reduction surgery. J Thorac Cardiovasc Surg 2012;143:47–54.e1.

24. Pompeo E, Mineo TC. Awake pulmonary metastasectomy. J Thorac Cardiovasc Surg 2007;133: 960–6.

25. Pompeo E, Tacconi F, Mineo D, et al. The role of awake video-assisted thoracoscopic surgery in spontaneous pneumothorax. J Thorac Cardiovasc Surg 2007;133:786–90.

26. Galvez C, Navarro-Martinez J, Bolufer S, et al. Awake non-intubated single-incision VATS lobectomy after induction chemotherapy and mediastinoscopy. Indian J Thorac Cardiovasc Surg 2018;34(1):69–72.

27. Pompeo E, Mineo TC. Awake operative videothoracoscopic pulmonary resections. Thorac Surg Clin 2008;18:311–20.

28. Noda M, Okada Y, Maeda S, et al. Is there a benefit of awake thoracoscopic surgery in patients with secondary spontaneous pneumothorax? J Thorac Cardiovasc Surg 2012;143:613–6.

29. Chen J, Cheng Y, Hung M, et al. Nonintubated thoracoscopic lobectomy for lung cancer. Ann Surg 2011;254:1038–43.

30. Liu J, Cui F, Li S, et al. Nonintubated video-assisted thoracoscopic surgery under epidural anesthesia compared with conventional anesthetic option: a randomized control study. Surg Innov 2015;22: 123–30.

31. Irons JF, Martinez G. Anaesthetic considerations for non-intubated thoracic surgery. J Vis Surg 2016;2: 61.

32. Shi Y, Yu H, Huang L, et al. Postoperative pulmonary complications and hospital stay after lung resection surgery: a metaanalysis comparing nonintubated and intubated anesthesia. Medicine (Baltimore) 2018;97(21):e10596.

33. Irons J, Miles L, Joshi K, et al. Intubated versus non-intubated general anesthesia for video-assisted thoracoscopic surgery: a case-control study. J Cardiothorac Vasc Anesth 2017;31:411–7.

34. Liu J, Cui F, Pompeo E, et al. The impact of nonintubated versus intubated anaesthesia on early outcomes of video-assisted thoracoscopic anatomical resection in non-small-cell lung cancer: a propensity score matching analysis. Eur J Cardiothorac Surg 2016;50:920–5.

35. Wu C, Chen J, Lin Y, et al. Feasibility and safety of nonintubated thoracoscopic lobectomy for geriatric lung cancer patients. Ann Thorac Surg 2013;95: 405–11.

36. Ramsay M, Savege T, Simpson B, et al. Controlled sedation with alphaxalone-alphadolone. Br Med J 1974;2:656–9.

37. Ms MH, Cheng Y, Chan K, et al. Nonintubated uniportal thoracoscopic surgery for peripheral lung nodules. Ann Thorac Surg 2014;98:1998–2003.

38. Hung M, Chan K, Liu Y, et al. Nonintubated thoracoscopic lobectomy for lung cancer using epidural anesthesia and intercostal blockade. Medicine (Baltimore) 2015;94:1–8.

39. Shao W, Phan K, Guo X, et al. Non-intubated complete thoracoscopic bronchial sleeve resection for central lung cancer. J Thorac Dis 2014;6: 1485–8.

40. Klijian A, Gibbs M, Andonian N. AVATS: awake video assisted thoracic surgery–extended series report. J Cardiothorac Surg 2014;9:149.

41. Wang M-L, Galvez C, Chen J-S, et al. Non-intubated single-incision video-assisted thoracic surgery: a two-center cohort of 188 patients. J Thorac Dis 2017;9:2587–98.

42. Kiss G, Castillo M. Non-intubated anesthesia in thoracic surgery — technical issues. Ann Transl Med 2015;3(8):109.

43. Matsumoto I, Oda M, Watanabe G. Awake endoscopic thymectomy via an infrasternal approach using sternal lifting. Thorac Cardiovasc Surg 2008;56: 311–3.

44. Al-abdullatief M, Wahood A, Al-shirawi N, et al. Awake anaesthesia for major thoracic surgical procedures: an observational study. Eur J Cardiothorac Surg 2007;32:346–50.

45. Elia S, Guggino G, Mineo D, et al. Awake one stage bilateral thoracoscopic sympathectomy for palmar hyperhidrosis: a safe outpatient procedure. Eur J Cardiothorac Surg 2005;28:312–7.

46. Galvez C, Navarro-Martinez J, Bolufer S, et al. Nonintubated uniportal left-lower lobe upper segmentectomy (S6). J Vis Surg 2017;3:48.

47. Galvez C, Bolufer S, Navarro-Martinez J, et al. Awake uniportal video-assisted thoracoscopic metastasectomy after a nasopharyngeal carcinoma. J Thorac Cardiovasc Surg 2014;147:e24–6.

48. David P, Pompeo E, Fabbi E, et al. Surgical pneumo-thorax under spontaneous ventilation — effect on oxygenation and ventilation. Ann Transl Med 2015; 3(8):106.

49. Galvez C, Navarro-Martinez J, Bolufer S, et al. Benefits of awake uniportal pulmonary resection in a patient with a previous contralateral lobectomy. Ann Transl Med 2014;2(9):93.

50. Gonzalez-Rivas D, Fernandez R, De la Torre M, et al. Single-port thoracoscopic lobectomy in a nonintubated patient: the least invasive procedure for major lung resection? Interact Cardiovasc Thorac Surg 2014;19:552–5.

51. Mineo TC, Tacconi F. From " awake " to " monitored anesthesia care " thoracic surgery: a 15 year evolution. Thorac Cancer 2014;5:1–13.

52. Rocco G, Romano V, Accardo R, et al. Awake single-access (uniportal) video-assisted thoracoscopic surgery for peripheral pulmonary nodules in a complete ambulatory setting. Ann Thorac Surg 2010;89: 1625–7.

53. Galvez C, Bolufer S, Navarro-Martinez J, et al. Non-intubated video-assisted thoracic surgery management of secondary spontaneous pneumothorax. Ann Transl Med 2015;3(8):104.

54. Rocco G. Non-intubated uniportal lung surgery. Eur J Cardiothorac Surg 2016;49(Suppl 1):i3–5.

55. Navarro-Martínez J, Gálvez C, Rivera-cogollos MJ, et al. Intraoperative crisis resource management during a non-intubated video-assisted thoracoscopic surgery. Ann Transl Med 2015;3(8):111.

56. Chen K, Cheng Y, Hung M, et al. Nonintubated thoracoscopic lung resection: a 3-year experience with 285 cases in a single institution. J Thorac Dis 2012;4:347–51.

57. Liu J, Cui F, He J. Non-intubated video-assisted thoracoscopic surgery anatomical resections: a new perspective for treatment of lung cancer. Chin J Cancer Res 2015;27:197–202.

58. Hung MH, Hsu H, Chen KC, et al. Nonintubated thoracoscopic anatomical segmentectomy for lung tumors. Ann Thorac Surg 2013;96:1209–15.

59. Guo Z, Shao W, Yin W, et al. Analysis of feasibility and safety of complete video-assisted thoracoscopic resection of anatomic pulmonary segments under non-intubated anesthesia. J Thorac Dis 2014;6:37–44.

60. Mineo TC, Tamburrini A, Perroni G, et al. One thousand cases of tubeless video-assisted thoracic surgery at the Rome Tor Vergata University. Future Oncol 2016;12(23s):13–8.

Video-Assisted Thoracoscopic Surgery Lobectomy for Lung Cancer in Nonintubated Anesthesia

Wan-Ting Hung, MD[a], Ya-Jung Cheng, MD, PhD[b],
Jin-Shing Chen, MD, PhD[c],*

KEYWORDS

- Video-assisted thoracoscopic surgery • Lung cancer • Nonintubated VATS • Awake VATS
- Regional anesthesia • Lobectomy

KEY POINTS

- Nonintubated video-assisted thoracoscopic surgery (VATS) lobectomy is a feasible and safe alternative for lung cancer treatment.
- A variety of anesthetic techniques have been reported, and methods for managing the airway, analgesia, and sedation should be considered separately.
- Surgical techniques used for nonintubated VATS lobectomy are similar to those of the intubated approach.
- In the case of conversion, anesthesiologists should be familiar with bronchoscopic-guided intubation in the lateral decubitus position, although the reported incidence of conversion is low.
- Nonintubated VATS lobectomy may provide the benefits of faster postoperative recovery and fewer intubation-related complications, but oncologic outcomes have not been reported.

INTRODUCTION

The development of video-assisted thoracoscopic surgery (VATS) lobectomy using a nonintubation technique in the past decade has marked a new beginning for thoracic surgery. One century ago, before the introduction of endotracheal intubation and positive pressure ventilation, creating large openings in the chest wall, which causes pulmonary collapse, was considered fatal. Thoracic surgery was limited to chest wall procedures and drainage of pleural effusion because of the "pneumothorax problem."[1] At that time, pulmonary lobectomy was associated with a high mortality and was mostly indicated for infectious diseases, such as bronchiectasis and tuberculosis.[2] The development of 1-stage lobectomy is considered to have begun with the work of Harold Brunn in 1929.[3] In his case series that included 5 bronchiectasis cases and 1 lung malignancy case, Brunn described the details of lobectomy using local anesthesia and morphine preceded by barbital; he also mentioned the importance of cough suppression and keeping the diaphragm

---

Disclosure Statement: The authors have nothing to disclose.
[a] Division of Thoracic Surgery, Department of Surgery, National Taiwan University Hospital, No. 7, Chung-Shan South Road, Taipei 10002, Taiwan; [b] Department of Anesthesiology, National Taiwan University Hospital, National Taiwan University College of Medicine, No. 7, Chung-Shan South Road, Taipei 10002, Taiwan; [c] Division of Thoracic Surgery, Department of Surgery, National Taiwan University Hospital and National Taiwan University College of Medicine, No. 7, Chung-Shan South Road, Taipei 10002, Taiwan
* Corresponding author.
E-mail address: chenjs@ntu.edu.tw

Thorac Surg Clin 30 (2020) 73–82
https://doi.org/10.1016/j.thorsurg.2019.09.002
1547-4127/20/© 2019 Elsevier Inc. All rights reserved.

quiet during the procedure. All 6 patients survived the perioperative course, but 1 patient died of malignancy 9 months after surgery. This report was one of the earliest reports of "nonintubated" pulmonary lobectomy.

In the 1930s, the application of a cuffed endotracheal tube with controlled ventilation led to a substantial revolution in the field and enabled deeper anesthesia to eliminate spontaneous respiration of the patients and provide a quiet surgical field.[4] During the following decades, advances were made in airway management, 1-lung ventilation, and mechanical ventilators; in addition, invasive and noninvasive intraoperative monitoring, the introduction of multiple anesthetic agents, and an understanding of pulmonary physiology and anatomy have contributed to the evolution of anesthesia for thoracic surgery. Intubated general anesthesia with 1-lung ventilation is considered the standard for thoracic surgery, and lung cancer has surpassed infectious diseases as the main indication for lobectomy. The advent of VATS began another revolution in thoracic surgery, and the first VATS lobectomy was reported in 1992.[5] As surgeons continued developing other minimally invasive techniques during the modern era, Pompeo and colleagues,[6] in 2004, first proposed the resection of pulmonary nodules by awake VATS without endotracheal intubation to prevent intubation-related complications and ventilator-induced lung injury. In 2007, Al-Abdullatief and colleagues[7] reported a retrospective observational study of awake anesthesia for major thoracic surgeries, including 3 lobectomies. The detailed techniques of nonintubated VATS (NIVATS) lobectomy to treat lung cancer were first reported by Chen and colleagues[8] in 2011. Over the years, other groups have described modifications and a variety of analgesia strategies, including different types of airway management, analgesia, and sedation methods. In this work, the authors review current literature regarding the techniques and outcomes of NIVATS lobectomy to treat lung cancer, its unsolved problems, and its future prospects.

INDICATIONS AND CONTRAINDICATIONS

Patients considered suitable for NIVATS lobectomy for lung cancer have clinical stage I or stage II disease and a tumor smaller than 6 cm in diameter, without evidence of chest wall, diaphragm, or main bronchus involvement. Common contraindications are listed in **Table 1**[8–10]; these mainly include oncologically unsound conditions or conditions rendering the nonintubated procedure unsafe. Extensive pleural adhesion or previous thoracic surgery contraindicates neither VATS lobectomy nor the nonintubated approach.[9] Patients with poor pulmonary function at high risk for intubated general anesthesia are considered ideal candidates for the nonintubated approach for minor thoracic surgery.[11,12] Wang and colleagues[13] reported the feasibility of NIVATS lobectomy in patients with impaired pulmonary function. However, because extremely poor lung function (forced expiratory volume in 1 second [FEV_1] <30% or diffusing capacity of the lung for carbon monoxide [DLCO] <30%) is considered a contraindication for VATS lobectomy because of the possibility of postoperative respiratory failure,[9] these conditions are also regarded as contraindications for the nonintubated approach. Obesity is associated with higher respiratory rates and lower tidal volumes,[14] and obese patients are more likely to develop faster and deeper respiratory movements during nonintubated anesthesia. In a recent study by Hung and colleagues[15] that included 1025 NIVATS lung tumor resections, body mass index (BMI) ≥25 kg/m² was found to be a risk factor for conversion to intubation. In many studies, BMI greater than 30 was considered an exclusion criterion for NIVATS.[11,16–18]

Table 1	
Contraindications for nonintubated video-assisted thoracoscopic surgery lobectomy	
Contraindications for VATS Lobectomy	**Contraindications for Nonintubated Approach**
ASA score >3	Sleep apnea
Bleeding disorder	Unfavorable airway anatomy
FEV_1 <30%	High risks for gastric reflux
DLCO <30%	Underlying neurologic or mental disorders
Centrality of tumor if invading hilar structure(s)	BMI >30
Severe cardiopulmonary dysfunction	Known allergy to local anesthetics
	Expected extensive pleural adhesion
	Unstable asthma
	Spine deformities (if TEA is to be used)

Abbreviation: ASA, American Society of Anesthesiologists.

PREOPERATIVE ASSESSMENT

The medical history of the patient should be carefully reviewed. Diagnostic evaluation and staging of the oncologic status are routinely performed, including laboratory hemograms, chemistry and coagulation profiles, imaging of the chest and upper abdomen with contrast-enhanced computed tomography (CT), integrated whole-body PET /CT, bone scan, and imaging of the brain with MRI or CT. A pathologic diagnosis is made according to preoperative biopsy or intraoperative frozen section results. A pulmonary function test should be performed, and an echocardiogram is indicated if the patient reports related symptoms or is elderly. Factors predictive of difficult intubation, such as an unfavorable airway, should be evaluated before surgery. The surgical team, including the surgeon and anesthesiologist, should evaluate the patient and reach a consensus. The patient should be informed of the risks and benefits of the nonintubated approach.

ANESTHETIC TECHNIQUES
Airway Management

The most important concepts of "awake" or "nonintubated" VATS are avoidance of tracheal intubation and muscle relaxants and maintenance of spontaneous breathing. Choices for airway management during NIVATS include the following:

- Face mask: During early studies of NIVATS, a face mask was used to keep the oxygen saturation (SpO_2) higher than 90% during surgery.[6–8] No significant differences in the lowest detectable mean SpO_2 and peak end-tidal carbon dioxide in intubated and nonintubated groups were found. However, intraoperative hypoxemia was still a concern and may result in conversion to intubated general anesthesia.[8]
- Laryngeal mask airway (LMA): In 2012, Ambrogi and colleagues[19] first reported a preliminary experience with VATS for patients under general anesthesia and spontaneous breathing with LMA. Later, the same group presented the feasibility and safety of this technique for VATS resection of lung nodules.[20] No desaturation was noted, even for older patients with chronic obstructive pulmonary disease (COPD) or patients heavier than 100 kg. The benefits include the ability to use general anesthesia with inhalation anesthetics, thus permitting positive pressure ventilation if breathing depression develops,

and the ability to use LMA-aided tracheal intubation to obtain an endotracheal airway if conversion is indicated.
- High-flow nasal cannula (HFNC): HFNC with transnasal humidified rapid-insufflation ventilatory exchange with a flow rate of 20 L/m effectively increases the oxygen reserve and safety margin during NIVATS[21] (**Fig. 1**).
- Oropharyngeal cannula: Some groups prefer an oropharyngeal cannula with a tip that lies immediately above the vocal cords to effectively increase the oxygen concentration of inspired air.[22]

Locoregional Anesthesia

The most common techniques for analgesia during NIVATS lobectomy are thoracic epidural anesthesia (TEA) and intercostal nerve blocks (ICNB). To achieve a sensory block between T2-9 while maintaining diaphragm movement, the usual level of epidural catheter insertion is at T4-T6. However, the TEA technique is time consuming and technically demanding, and it may cause unwanted complications. An ICNB can be used to prevent TEA-related complications. Hung and colleagues[23] reported a retrospective cohort study of 238 cases that was performed to compare TEA and ICNB for NIVATS lobectomy for lung cancer; they found no difference in postoperative analgesia. ICNB can be performed easily and quickly, does not cause hemodynamic instability, and does not create a risk for spinal cord injury. Usually, local anesthetic agents are infiltrated under direct thoracoscopic vision from the third to the eighth intercostal nerves after creation of the first thoracoscopy port; bupivacaine is the most widely used (**Fig. 2**).

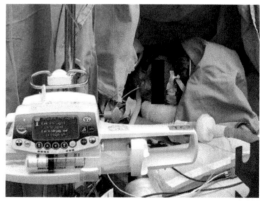

Fig. 1. Anesthetic settings of nonintubated thoracoscopic surgery. The patient was sedated with propofol and breathed through an HFNC.

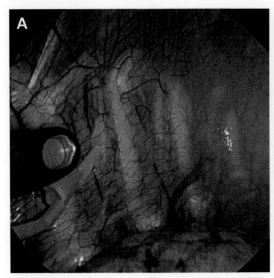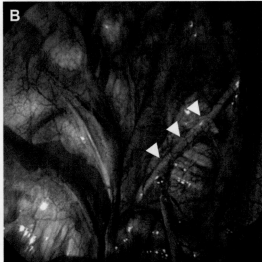

Fig. 2. (*A*) ICNB and (*B*) right-sided vagal block adjacent to the vagus nerve (*arrowheads*).

Sedation

The depth of sedation is a continuum in NIVATS, from mildly sedated but communicable and cooperative to a sedation level of general anesthesia. Whichever depth of sedation is applied, the patients should be monitored closely to ensure that they maintain a respiration rate between 12 and 20 breaths/min. NIVATS lobectomy can be performed with the patient awake, as reported by Al-Abdullatief and colleagues and Chen and colleagues.[7,8] However, to decrease patient anxiety and to provide a more stable and controlled surgical environment for surgeons, deeper sedation with target-controlled infusion of propofol and/or remifentanil and bispectral index monitoring to maintain a target of 40 to 60 is favored by most groups.[10,16–18,24,25] A bispectral index range of 40 to 60 corresponds to a hypnotic state of general anesthesia while spontaneous breathing is maintained. Some investigators used incremental or continuously infused remifentanil to slow the respiratory rate and suppress the cough reflex.[26,27] For patients with LMA for ventilation support, inhalatory agents, such as sevoflurane, can be used for analgesia instead of intravenous hypnotic drugs.

Cough Suppression and Vagal Nerve Block

VATS lobectomy involves bronchial manipulation, which may induce an unwanted cough reflex during nonintubated surgery. Dissection of vascular structures without cough control is not safe because of the risk of major bleeding. The cough reflex is controlled through either intrathoracic vagus nerve infiltration or preemptive inhalation of nebulized lidocaine 2% for 30 minutes before surgery. However, because vagal block is effective for diminishing the cough reflex, easy to perform, and associated with low risks, it is the authors' preferred option. Vagal block is usually performed with intrathoracic administration of 2 to 3 mL 0.5% bupivacaine to the vagus nerve at the level of the lower trachea for right-sided procedures and at the level of the aortopulmonary window for left-sided procedures (see **Fig. 2**).[8]

SURGICAL TECHNIQUES

The surgical setting for NIVATS lobectomy is similar to that for intubated VATS lobectomy. Patients are placed in the lateral decubitus position. Traditionally, VATS lobectomy is performed using a 3-port method, as described by McKenna.[28] After creation of the first skin incision under local anesthesia, the lung is collapsed gradually to enable further application of ICNB or intrathoracic vagal block. Further procedures are consistent with those of conventional VATS (**Fig. 3**). Systemic lymph node dissection includes more than 3 stations of the mediastinal lymph nodes. When the procedure has been completed, manually assisted mask ventilation is provided to reexpand the lung after closure of the surgical wounds with sutures. Alternatively, if the patient is oxygenated with an HFNC, then a high flow of oxygen at 70 L/min can be provided; if an LMA is used, then positive pressure ventilation can be applied. Suction via the chest tube can also be used to help lung expansion.

In 2014, Gonzalez-Rivas and colleagues[29] reported the first single-port NIVATS lobectomy

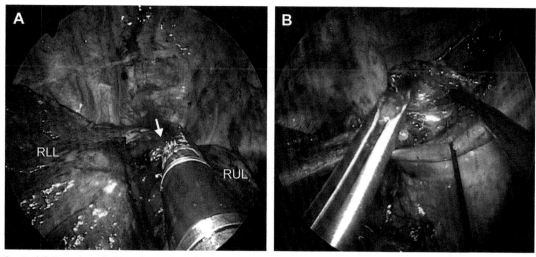

Fig. 3. (*A*) Bronchus division (*arrow*) and (*B*) pretracheal lymph node dissection during a nonintubated thoracoscopic right upper lobectomy. RLL, right lower lobe; RUL, right upper lobe.

and ushered the concept of minimally invasive thoracoscopic surgery into a new era. Local intercostal anesthesia was applied without epidural anesthesia or vagal blockade in their case. LMA with sevoflurane gas was used, and a target-controlled infusion of remifentanil was administered. The patient was discharged home 36 hours after the procedure. Other groups also demonstrated the feasibility and satisfactory early postoperative outcomes of uniportal NIVATS lobectomy.[17,18,30] Although more evidence is necessary to clarify the risks and benefits of this advancement, nonintubated uniportal VATS lobectomy is probably the least invasive approach to lung cancer surgery.

MANAGEMENT OF SPECIAL CONDITIONS
Hypercapnia and Hypoxemia

For patients undergoing NIVATS, respiratory function under spontaneous ventilation is concerning. Intraoperative hypercapnia may develop gradually, but the change is usually tolerable and transient.[31,32] When necessary, it can be corrected with manual mask ventilation. Partial pressure of carbon dioxide ($Paco_2$) usually gradually returns to normal after wound closure. During nonintubated surgery, perfusion of the dependent lung is better than intubated general anesthesia because of negative pressure in the dependent lung and increased pulmonary vascular resistance of the operated lung. Therefore, oxygenation may be better with NIVATS. In the case of hypoxemia, the HFNC and LMA may provide better oxygenation than a simple face mask.[21] However, when

intractable hypoxemia develops during 1-lung ventilation, conversion to tracheal intubation may be required.

Conversion to Tracheal Intubation

The most common reason for conversion to intubated general anesthesia is significant mediastinal movement.[15] Although in most patients the surgical pneumothorax is well tolerated and the operated lung remains motionless, some patients develop significant respiratory movement. Obesity is considered a risk factor. Other common causes for conversion are listed in **Table 2**.[8,15–18,23–25,27] Although conversion to intubated general anesthesia is considered a technically demanding procedure for anesthesiologists, only a few situations are urgent, such as major bleeding, and the reported incidence is low (0.4%–3%).[15,16,25] When this occurs, the surgeon must first control the bleeding, while the anesthesiologist intubates the patient in the lateral decubitus position under the guidance of a bronchoscope within a few minutes. Most conditions warranting conversion are elective and nonurgent, and surgeons and anesthesiologists may feel less stress and have more time to prepare for conversion. Surgical wounds can be sealed with transparent waterproof dressings after placement of a chest tube to reexpand the collapsed lung and to improve oxygenation before intubation. Therefore, surgeons should be aware of intraoperative conditions that may result in emergency situations, such as dissecting a dense hilar adhesion or calcified lymph nodes.

Table 2
Reasons for conversion to intubated general anesthesia

Emergency Situations	Elective Situations Related to Surgery Safety	Elective Situations Related to Anesthesia Safety
Hemodynamic instability	Lack of progress during surgery related to the surgeon's experience	Hypercapnia
	Vigorous mediastinal or diaphragmatic movement	Acidosis
	Intractable cough	Failure of regional nerve block
	Tumor invasion	

POSTOPERATIVE CARE

In general, postoperative care for NIVATS lobectomy is similar to that for intubated lobectomy. Because muscle relaxants are not used and there is no tracheal intubation, patients can resume oral intake 2 to 4 hours after surgery. Postoperative analgesics consist of oral analgesics and incremental intravenous analgesics or continuous epidural anesthesia. Chest radiography is performed immediately postoperatively or the next morning, depending on the individual protocol at each hospital. The chest tube can be removed if no air leaks are present and if the drainage amount is less than 200 mL during a 24-hour period.

ANESTHETIC AND SURGICAL OUTCOMES
Safety and Feasibility

Two meta-analyses have been conducted to compare the short-term feasibility and safety of nonintubated thoracic surgery with those of intubated VATS, and the results showed significantly shorter hospital stays and fewer postoperative complications for nonintubated patients.[33,34] Although not many groups have reported experiences with NIVATS lobectomy, the available literature demonstrated the safety and feasibility of NIVATS lobectomy. Five studies that compared NIVATS lobectomy with intubated VATS lobectomy indicated that the anesthetic induction time, operative time, and intraoperative blood loss were all comparable in both groups, and no in-hospital mortality was reported in these studies (**Table 3**).[8,16,25,35,36] The risk for conversion to tracheal intubation was between 0% and 15%, and the rate of conversion to thoracotomy was approximately 3%.

Benefits

In general, the benefits of NIVATS lobectomy are its faster postoperative recovery times and fewer intubation-related complications. Three comparative studies showed significantly shorter postoperative fasting times for NIVATS lobectomy than for intubated VATS lobectomy.[8,25,35] Two studies showed significantly less postoperative pleural drainage and shorter postoperative hospital stays.[25,35] Patients in the nonintubated group also had significantly lower rates of sore throats, less need for nasogastric tube insertion, and shorter durations of postoperative antibiotic use.[8,35]

Surgical stress is also reduced after nonintubated surgery. Awake VATS results in attenuated stress hormone release, decreased postoperative C-reactive protein peaks, and reduced lymphocyte responses compared with equivalent procedures performed using intubated VATS for nononcologic thoracic disease.[37,38] Another study performed by Liu and colleagues[35] indicated that NIVATS was associated with a lower level of inflammatory cytokines in bronchioalveolar lavage fluid and serum for bullae surgery. Although data and clinical relevance are not available for lobectomy, NIVATS appears to be a possible method to decrease the inflammatory changes owing to 1-lung ventilation and positive pressure-related trauma.

Oncologic Treatment Efficacy

Most studies found that the numbers of dissected lymph nodes were comparable in the NIVATS and intubated VATS lobectomy groups.[8,25,35,36] However, 1 study by AlGhamdi and colleagues[16] showed that significantly fewer lymph nodes were retrieved from the nonintubated group. Data regarding long-term oncologic outcomes, such as survival, are not yet available. Therefore, further studies are warranted to clarify the oncologic adequacy of this innovative technique.

Table 3
Comparative studies of awake and nonintubated video-assisted thoracoscopic surgery lobectomy performed by different groups

First Author, Year	Study Period	Study Type	No. of NIVATS/IVATS Patients	Age, Year (NIVATS/IVATS)[a]	Preoperative BMI (NIVATS/IVATS)[a]	Preoperative FEV$_1$ of (NIVATS/IVATS)[a]	Airway Management	Locoregional Analgesia	Sedation Drug	Mean Blood Loss, mL	Postoperative Fasting Time, h	Postoperative Hospital Stays, d	NIVATS Conversion to IVATS, %	Complications, % (NIVATS/IVATS)	Other Outcomes of NIVATS
Chen et al,[8] 2011	August 2009–June 2010	Retrospective comparative	30/30	57.9 ± 10.4/56.5 ± 9.5	24.0 ± 3.2/23.4 ± 3.3	105.1 ± 17.9/104.3 ± 12.2	Face mask	TEA	Propofol	125.8/166.8	4.7/18.8 (P<.001[b])	5.9 ± 2.2/7.1 ± 3.2	10	13.3/36.7	Fewer postoperative sore throat cases and NG tube insertions
Wu et al,[36] 2013	September 2009–December 2011	Retrospective comparative	36/48	72.9 (65–84)/73.0 (65–87)	23.2 ± 2.1/23.9 ± 2.7	112.8 ± 26.4/106.1 ± 23.5	Face mask	TEA	Propofol	160.6/167.5	—	6.7 ± 3.3/7.2 ± 3.5	2.8	25/35	Shorter induction times, higher peak PaCO$_2$ values for 1-lung ventilation
Liu et al,[35] 2015	July 2011–July 2012	Randomized controlled	26/30	56.2/56.2	—	—	NP airway, LMA, or face mask	TEA	Remifentanil, propofol	250.2/156.3	10.8/17.7 (P<.001[b])	9.5/12.7 (P=.022[b])	15.4	6.7/16.7	Less postoperative antibiotic use, less postoperative pleural drainage
Liu et al,[25] 2016	December 2011–December 2014	Retrospective propensity score-matching	116/116	56.0 ± 10.3/57.3 ± 10.5	22.4 ± 2.5/22.5 ± 3.43	—	—	TEA	Remifentanil, propofol	124.4/142.6	6.7/12.3 (P<.001[b])	7.4 ± 2.0/8.6 ± 4.1 (P=.035[b])	7.0	8.6/10.3	Less postoperative pleural drainage
AlGhamdi et al,[16] 2018	January 2016–December 2016	Retrospective comparative	30/30	64.9 ± 10.5/66.1 ± 9.5	23.8 ± 3.2/23.5 ± 2.9	94.8 ± 9.3/95.1 ± 16.8	Face mask	ICNB	Propofol and dexmedetomidate	82.3/78.3	—	6.9 ± 3.8/7.6 ± 5.3	3	20/20	Fewer dissected lymph nodes

Abbreviations: —, not mentioned; BIS, bispectral index; IVATS, intubated video-assisted thoracoscopic surgery; NG, nasogastric; NP, nasopharyngeal.
[a] Continuous data are shown as mean ± standard deviation or median (range).
[b] P<.05 is statistically significant.

SPECIAL CONSIDERATIONS FOR HIGH-RISK GROUPS
Patients with Impaired Lung Function

Patients with impaired lung function or COPD are considered to be at a high risk for intubated general anesthesia. Previous studies have demonstrated the feasibility and improved recovery of awake thoracic surgery for patients with severely impaired lung function undergoing lung volume reduction surgery or lung biopsy.[12,39,40] Furthermore, Wang and colleagues[13] reported 28 patients with FEV_1 less than 70% who underwent NIVATS for lung tumor resection. Among them, 18 patients had primary lung cancer and 4 patients underwent lobectomy. One patient required conversion to intubated 1-lung ventilation because of persistent intraoperative wheezing and labored breathing. Overall, 5 patients developed prolonged air leaks; 2 patients developed acute exacerbations of COPD, and 1 patient developed new-onset atrial fibrillation postoperatively. The preliminary study showed the technical feasibility of NIVATS for lung tumor resections, including lobectomy, for patients with impaired lung function. However, because of the small patient number, more evidence is required to confirm the safety.

Elderly Patients

A retrospective study by Wu and colleagues[36] that compared NIVATS lobectomy with intubated lobectomy for geriatric patients with lung cancer (65 years or older) indicated that the nonintubated group had shorter anesthetic induction times, less intravenous fluid administration, and comparable lowest intraoperative SpO_2 levels. The peak $PaCO_2$ during 1-lung ventilation was significantly higher for nonintubated patients than for intubated patients, but the hemodynamics was well maintained, and hypercapnia resolved soon after surgery. Operative time, blood loss, and postoperative complications, such as prolonged air leaks, pneumonia, vomiting, and cardiac complications, were comparable in both groups. This study demonstrated that NIVATS lobectomy is a valid alternative for managing geriatric patients with lung cancer.

Although studies have shown the feasibility and safety of NIVATS lobectomy for these high-risk groups, the authors suggest that surgical teams should accumulate more experience performing NIVATS lobectomy for low-risk groups before applying this technique to high-risk groups.

UNSOLVED PROBLEMS AND RECOMMENDATIONS FOR FUTURE RESEARCH

In the past decade, anesthesiologists and surgeons revisited the feasibility and safety of VATS lobectomy without tracheal intubation for lung cancer. However, the evidence of its benefits is not strong enough because of the lack of prospective, randomized, controlled studies. The diversity of the anesthetic techniques and surgical procedures also made it difficult to compare the results of different studies. Although the adverse effects of tracheal intubation and ventilator-associated lung injury have been recognized, it is still difficult to compare the tradeoffs between the benefits and risks of nonintubated and intubated VATS lobectomy. Furthermore, long-term oncologic results to clarify the adequacy of VATS lobectomy for cancer treatment are still awaited. The following research directions would help to solve these problems:

- Well-designed, prospective, randomized, controlled studies of patients with lung cancer treated with nonintubated or intubated VATS lobectomy.
- Studies that provide mid-term or long-term oncologic outcomes of NIVATS lobectomy.
- Studies that determine more biomarkers or measurable physiologic outcomes that can reveal the potential benefits and clinical significance of the nonintubated approach.

SUMMARY

NIVATS lobectomy is a feasible and safe alternative for lung cancer treatment, and it may be used for high-risk patients, such as those with impaired lung function or elderly patients. Its benefits include faster postoperative recovery and fewer intubation-related complications. However, long-term oncologic outcomes have not been reported. Future prospective, randomized, controlled studies should be performed to obtain more evidence regarding the benefits and risks of NIVATS lobectomy.

REFERENCES

1. Matas R. Intralaryngeal Insufflation. For the relief of acute surgical pneumothorax. Its history and methods with a description of the latest devices for this purpose. JAMA 1900;23:1468–73.
2. Lindskog GE. A history of pulmonary resection. Yale J Biol Med 1957;30:187–200.
3. Brunn H. Surgical principles underlying one-stage lobectomy. Arch Surg 1929;18:490–515.

4. Brodsky JB, Lemmens HJ. The history of anesthesia for thoracic surgery. Minerva Anestesiol 2007;73: 513–24.

5. Landreneau RJ, Mack MJ, Hazelrigg SR, et al. Video-assisted thoracic surgery: basic technical concepts and intercostal approach strategies. Ann Thorac Surg 1992;54:800–7.

6. Pompeo E, Mineo D, Rogliani P, et al. Feasibility and results of awake thoracoscopic resection of solitary pulmonary nodules. Ann Thorac Surg 2004;78: 1761–8.

7. Al-Abdullatief M, Wahood A, Al-Shirawi N, et al. Awake anaesthesia for major thoracic surgical procedures: an observational study. Eur J Cardiothorac Surg 2007;32:346–50.

8. Chen JS, Cheng YJ, Hung MH, et al. Nonintubated thoracoscopic lobectomy for lung cancer. Ann Surg 2011;254:1038–43.

9. Yan TD, Cao C, D'Amico TA, et al. Video-assisted thoracoscopic surgery lobectomy at 20 years: a consensus statement. Eur J Cardiothorac Surg 2014;45:633–9.

10. Moon Y, AlGhamdi ZM, Jeon J, et al. Non-intubated thoracoscopic surgery: initial experience at a single center. J Thorac Dis 2018;10:3490–8.

11. Pompeo E, Sorge R, Akopov A, et al. Non-intubated thoracic surgery–a survey from the European Society of Thoracic Surgeons. Ann Transl Med 2015;3:37.

12. Kiss G, Claret A, Desbordes J, et al. Thoracic epidural anaesthesia for awake thoracic surgery in severely dyspnoeic patients excluded from general anaesthesia. Interact Cardiovasc Thorac Surg 2014;19:816–23.

13. Wang ML, Hung MH, Hsu HH, et al. Non-intubated thoracoscopic surgery for lung cancer in patients with impaired pulmonary function. Ann Transl Med 2019;7:40.

14. Littleton SW. Impact of obesity on respiratory function. Respirology 2012;17:43–9.

15. Hung WT, Hung MH, Wang ML, et al. Nonintubated thoracoscopic surgery for lung tumor: seven years' experience with 1025 cases. Ann Thorac Surg 2019;107:1607–12.

16. AlGhamdi M, Lynhiavu L, Moon Y, et al. Comparison of non-intubated versus intubated video-assisted thoracoscopic lobectomy for lung cancer. J Thorac Dis 2018;10:4236–43.

17. Ahn S, Moon Y, AlGhamdi ZM, et al. Nonintubated uniportal video-assisted thoracoscopic surgery: a single-center experience. Korean J Thorac Cardiovasc Surg 2018;51:344–9.

18. Furák J, Szabó Z, Horváth T, et al. Non-intubated, uniportal, video assisted thoracic surgery [VATS] lobectomy, as a new procedure in our department. Magy Seb 2017;70:113–7 [in Hungarian].

19. Ambrogi MC, Fanucchi O, Gemignani R, et al. Video-assisted thoracoscopic surgery with spontaneous breathing laryngeal mask anesthesia: preliminary experience. J Thorac Cardiovasc Surg 2012;144: 514–5.

20. Ambrogi MC, Fanucchi O, Korasidis S, et al. Nonintubated thoracoscopic pulmonary nodule resection under spontaneous breathing anesthesia with laryngeal mask. Innovations (Phila) 2014;9:276–80.

21. Wang ML, Hung MH, Chen JS, et al. Nasal high-flow oxygen therapy improves arterial oxygenation during one-lung ventilation in non-intubated thoracoscopic surgery. Eur J Cardiothorac Surg 2018;53: 1001–6.

22. Galvez C, Navarro-Martinez J, Bolufer S, et al. Nonintubated uniportal VATS pulmonary anatomical resections. J Vis Surg 2017;3:120.

23. Hung MH, Chan KC, Liu YJ, et al. Nonintubated thoracoscopic lobectomy for lung cancer using epidural anesthesia and intercostal blockade. Medicine 2015;94:e727.

24. Hung MH, Hsu HH, Chan KC, et al. Non-intubated thoracoscopic surgery using internal intercostal nerve block, vagal block and targeted sedation. Eur J Cardiothorac Surg 2014;46:620–5.

25. Liu J, Cui F, Pompeo E, et al. The impact of non-intubated versus intubated anaesthesia on early outcomes of video-assisted thoracoscopic anatomical resection in non-small-cell lung cancer: a propensity score matching analysis. Eur J Cardiothorac Surg 2016;50:920–5.

26. Inoue K, Moriyama K, Takeda J. Remifentanil for awake thoracoscopic bullectomy. J Cardiothorac Vasc Anesth 2010;24:386–7.

27. Gonzalez-Rivas D, Bonome C, Fieira E, et al. Non-intubated video-assisted thoracoscopic lung resections: the future of thoracic surgery? Eur J Cardiothorac Surg 2016;49:721–31.

28. McKenna R. Lobectomy by video-assisted thoracic surgery with mediastinal node sampling for lung cancer. J Thorac Cardiovasc Surg 1994;107:879–82.

29. Gonzalez-Rivas D, Fernandez R, de la Torre M, et al. Single-port thoracoscopic lobectomy in a nonintubated patient: the least invasive procedure for major lung resection? Interact Cardiovasc Thorac Surg 2014;19:552–5.

30. Gonzalez-Rivas D, Yang Y, Guido W, et al. Non-intubated (tubeless) uniportal video-assisted thoracoscopic lobectomy. Ann Cardiothorac Surg 2016;5: 151–3.

31. Dong Q, Liang L, Li Y, et al. Anesthesia with nontracheal intubation in thoracic surgery. J Thorac Dis 2012;4:126–30.

32. Liu YJ, Hung MH, Hsu HH, et al. Effects on respiration of nonintubated anesthesia in thoracoscopic surgery under spontaneous ventilation. Ann Transl Med 2015;3:107.

33. Bertolaccini L, Zaccagna G, Divisi D, et al. Awake non-intubated thoracic surgery: an attempt of

systematic review and meta-analysis. Video Assist Thorac Surg 2017;2:59.

34. Deng HY, Zhu ZJ, Wang YC, et al. Non-intubated video-assisted thoracoscopic surgery under loco-regional anaesthesia for thoracic surgery: a meta-analysis. Interact Cardiovasc Thorac Surg 2016;23: 31–40.

35. Liu J, Cui F, Li S, et al. Nonintubated video-assisted thoracoscopic surgery under epidural anesthesia compared with conventional anesthetic option. Surg Innov 2015;22:123–30.

36. Wu CY, Chen JS, Lin YS, et al. Feasibility and safety of nonintubated thoracoscopic lobectomy for geriatric lung cancer patients. Ann Thorac Surg 2013; 95:405–11.

37. Vanni G, Tacconi F, Sellitri F, et al. Impact of awake videothoracoscopic surgery on postoperative lymphocyte responses. Ann Thorac Surg 2010;90:973–8.

38. Tacconi F, Pompeo E, Sellitri F, et al. Surgical stress hormones response is reduced after awake videothoracoscopy. Interact Cardiovasc Thorac Surg 2010;10:666–71.

39. Pompeo E, Tacconi F, Mineo TC. Comparative results of non-resectional lung volume reduction performed by awake or non-awake anesthesia. Eur J Cardiothorac Surg 2011;39:e51–8.

40. Pompeo E, Rogliani P, Tacconi F, et al. Randomized comparison of awake nonresectional versus nonawake resectional lung volume reduction surgery. J Thorac Cardiovasc Surg 2012;143:47–54.e1.

Nonintubated Anesthesia for Tracheal/Carinal Resection and Reconstruction

Hengrui Liang, MD[a,1], Diego Gonzalez-Rivas, MD[b,1], Yanran Zhou, MD[c,1],
Jun Liu, MD, PhD[a], Xi Wu, MD[c], Jianxing He, MD, PhD[a,*],
Shuben Li, MD, PhD[a,*]

KEYWORDS

• Nonintubated anesthesia • Tracheal/carinal resection • Reconstruction

KEY POINTS

• Nonintubated anesthesia is feasible and might be associated with shorter surgery time and shorter hospitalization for tracheal/carinal resection and reconstruction.
• Only case reports and a few small retrospective series study were conducted to evaluate nonintubated anesthesia for tracheal/carinal resection and reconstruction; no randomized control trials exist.
• Further exploration should focus on selection of optimal candidates and prospective validation.

BACKGROUND

Tracheal resection with end-to-end anastomosis is a very frequent intervention for tracheal tumor or stenosis in general. Tracheal tumor is a rare tumor of the upper respiratory system, consisting of only 2% upper respiratory neoplasms.[1] It usually presents with airway obstruction and irritating symptoms, including cough, sore throat, dyspnea, and shortness of breath. The diagnosis of such disease is confirmed by fibrobronchoscopy or computed tomography. Tracheal stenosis may be caused by prolonged mechanical ventilation, intraluminal and extraluminal neoplasms, or trauma.[2] The resection of stenotic airway segments may significantly improve the patient's quality of life. However, anesthetic management for both tracheal neoplasms and stenosis procedures is challenging.[3]

Mechanically induced ventilation with intubated anesthesia is considered standard care during tracheal resection and anastomosis, including upper, intrathoracic, and carinal tumor, which requires careful coordination between the surgical and anesthesia teams during airway excision and anastomosis.[4] Once the trachea is transected, a second tube is inserted into the distal airway to assure ventilation. However, mechanically induced ventilation is widely associated with pulmonary damage, and endotracheal intubation also increases the risk of airway edema and stenosis.[5,6] In some special cases, the intubation could

Funding: (1) Application, industrialization and generalization of surgical incision protector (2011B090400589); (2) The application of spontaneous ventilation and uniportal in complex thoracic surgery (A2015049).

[a] Department of Thoracic Surgery, The First Affiliated Hospital of Guangzhou Medical University, State Key Laboratory of Respiratory Disease, National Clinical Research Center for Respiratory Disease, Guangzhou Institute of Respiratory Health, No.151 of Yanjiangxi Road, Yuexiu, Guangzhou, Guangdong, China; [b] Department of Thoracic Surgery, Coruña University Hospital, Xubias 84, Coruña 15006, Spain; [c] Department of Anesthesia, The First Affiliated Hospital of Guangzhou Medical University, No.151 of Yanjiangxi Road, Yuexiu, Guangzhou, Guangdong, China

[1] These authors contributed equally to this work.

* Corresponding authors.

E-mail addresses: drjianxing.he@gmail.com (J.H.); 13500030280@163.com (S.L.)

be challenging because of a narrowed airway; then, endoscopic dilation should be arranged, which may be less effective.

Spontaneous ventilation-induced nonintubated surgery has been intensively investigated recently and reported to reduce the perioperative adverse effects of tracheal intubation and general anesthesia in many thoracic diseases.[7–10] In addition, in order to maintain spontaneous ventilation, the nonintubated procedure is performed without or with very little muscle relaxant, which might be another factor contributing to more rapid recovery after surgery.[11] Furthermore, without the influence of the tracheal tube, end-to-end anastomosis of tracheal has become not only easier and faster but also tidier.[12]

Currently, the evidence on application of nonintubated anesthesia is mainly from case reports, and only 2 case series studies. In 2010, Macchiarini and colleagues[13] first reported a case series of 21 upper tracheal resections for benign stenosis in nonintubated awake patients. Cervical epidural anesthesia and awake sedation were used to maintain spontaneous breathing during surgery. No intraoperative intubation or jet ventilation was required. Twenty consecutive patients with subglottic or upper trachea stenosis were enrolled. Permissive hypercapnia was well tolerated perioperatively. There was no conversion to intubation during surgery or early complications. They experienced only 1 case that required a nasotracheal tube for 36 hours after the surgical procedure. Patients had excellent or good functional outcomes, with no early relapse of stenosis. The investigators suggested that awake and tubeless upper airway surgery is feasible and safe and has a high level of patient satisfaction.

Jiang and colleagues[14] in their surgical center then published the first propensity matching cohorts in 2018, demonstrating that spontaneous ventilation is a feasible procedure in airway surgery in highly selected patients. A total of 18 patients were collected in their study; patients with tracheal/carinal tumor were treated with traditional or spontaneous ventilation video-assisted thoracic surgery (VATS) resection and reconstruction. Both median operative time, carinal reconstruction, and tracheal end-to-end anastomosis times were significantly shorter in the spontaneous ventilation group compared with the intubated group. The lowest oxygen saturation during the procedure was similar in 2 cohorts. No conversion to tracheal intubation was needed in the spontaneous ventilation group. No difference was observed regarding postoperative complications in the 2 groups. Their study suggested that spontaneous ventilation surgery could be a valid alternative to conventional intubated VATS for airway surgery. They emphasized that nonintubated airway surgery not only avoids general anesthesia with tracheal intubation and mechanical ventilation but also provides an ideal surgical field without any intraoperative tubing systems. However, they also proposed 2 major shortages: the first was the small sample size with limited its repeatability in other cohorts, and the second was that strict restriction for body mass index (BMI) of less than 25 would affect its use in a larger population, for example, western countries.

Except for the above 2 case series studies, several case reports describe the use of nonintubated anesthesia in other tracheal surgeries. Shao and colleagues[15] reported a case of complete endoscopic bronchial sleeve resection of right lower lung cancer under nonintubated epidural anesthesia. Peng and colleagues[16] described the technique of nonintubated complete thoracoscopic surgery for carinal reconstruction in a patient with adenocarcinoma of the trachea. Guo and colleagues[17] introduced a case of uniportal video-assisted thoracoscopic surgery in tracheal tumor under spontaneous ventilation anesthesia. Caronia and colleagues[18] reported a cervical tracheal resection and reconstruction under spontaneous ventilation anesthesia. Because of the failure of the repeated endoscopic dilatations and severe stenosis, in their case, nonintubated surgery was the only strategy for a definitive management of tracheal stenosis.

Since the first attempt on nonintubated anesthesia for tracheal resection and reconstruction in 2014,[15] the authors' center has completed more than 50 such cases. In this study, the authors review this topic and provide some of their experiences on nonintubated anesthesia for tracheal/carinal resection and the reconstruction technique in their center.

ANESTHESIA MANAGEMENT
Preparation Before Anesthesia

Electrocardiogram, heart rate, percutaneous oxygen saturation (Spo_2), end-tidal carbon dioxide partial pressure, and noninvasive blood pressure were routinely monitored after the patient entered the operating room; midazolam and atropine were administered 30 minutes before anesthesia induction.

Anesthesia Induction and Maintenance

Tracheal reconstruction under spontaneous ventilation anesthesia was performed using intravenous anesthesia combined with regional nerve block according to the location and operation of the tracheal tumor, including bilateral superficial cervical plexus block, thoracic paravertebral nerve block, vagus nerve block, and phrenic nerve block.

A laryngeal mask airway (LMA) (Double-laryngeal mask [FORNIA, Disposable Laryngeal Mask]) was used as a supraglottic device for tracheal reconstruction under spontaneous ventilation anesthesia. The laryngeal mask can be easily placed without using a muscle relaxant. Without a muscle relaxant, the airway obstruction caused by the relaxation of the throat muscle is avoided. The LMA is suitable for patients with tracheal tumor or upper trachea stenosis, avoiding difficult tracheal intubation. Single-lumen tracheal tube or a blocked tube could go through the laryngeal mask during surgery for some special needs. The sealing pressure of the LMA can reach 40 cm H_2O, which meets the requirements of high ventilation resistance. Maintaining an unobstructed airway is the key to tracheal reconstruction under spontaneous ventilation anesthesia. Timely airway suction and distal tracheal suspension are beneficial for obtaining stable oxygenation after the airway is opened.

Cervical Tracheal Reconstruction

Cervical tracheal reconstruction is commonly used in patients with upper airway tumors or postintubation tracheal stenosis. Intravenous sedation and bilateral superficial cervical plexus block can provide adequate analgesia and maintain spontaneous breathing during the operation, and intratracheal anesthesia can avoid intraoperative cough reflexes. Cervical epidural anesthesia, which was selected for upper airway surgery in the previous studies, had been proven to possibly lead to fatal complications, including spinal block, epidural hematoma, bilateral nerve phrenic paralysis, and systemic hypotension.[19] Therefore, the authors prefer bilateral cervical superficial plexus block. According to their experience, after the trachea was opened, the oxygenation and hypercapnia would improve because of the removal of the airway obstruction. When the airway was divided, patients breathed air through the distal tracheal, maintaining Spo_2 greater than 90%. Mild hypercapnia was noted in some patients, caused by a decrease of minute volume during sedation.

Tracheal and Carinal Reconstruction

VATS tracheal and carinal resection and reconstruction under spontaneous ventilation anesthesia is stricter and more difficult than cervical tracheal reconstruction. Intravenous sedation

combined with thoracic paravertebral nerve block is also recommended. An oxygen tube would be placed in the distal trachea or the contralateral main bronchus via the incision after opening the airway. The contralateral lung retains spontaneous breathing to maintain oxygenation. Thoracoscopic vagal nerve block can be simply operated and effectively prevents intraoperative cough. If diaphragmatic movement is obvious during the operation, phrenic nerve block can be performed.

Hypercapnia is common during VATS tracheal and carinal resection and reconstruction. In the authors' experience, P_aCO_2 may increase to 80 mm Hg, but it never causes hemodynamics unstable and anesthesia conversion, which is also reported by Jiang and colleagues.[14]

Conversion to Intubation

Conversion to intubation at any time during surgery is feasible. According to the authors' experience, a decrease in Spo_2 occurs during the opening of the airway, and a high-frequency snorkel can be connected to the hollow main tube or the main bronchus. When using high-frequency ventilation, it should be confirmed that the airway is open to prevent air pressure or pneumothorax. If improvement of Spo_2 is not obvious, conversion to tracheal intubation should be performed.

SURGERY PROCESS
Upper Trachea Resection and Reconstruction

The authors have described the technique of upper trachea resection and reconstruction and reported a case in 2016.[20] The patient was placed in the standard supine position with dorsal flexion of the neck. Sedation was started; also, 40% to 50% oxygen was delivered using a laryngeal mask, and cardiorespiratory vital parameters were constantly monitored as mentioned before. To ensure surgical safety, devices for tracheal intubation and mechanical ventilation were readily available in case of life-threatening airway obstruction or other complications. An additional dose of 2% lidocaine was injected into the surgical site during the operation to achieve an adequate level of anesthesia. At the time of skin incision, lidocaine was infiltrated in the cervical incision area (**Fig. 1**). Dissection was carried out in a standard way, and, after identification of the upper airway, the trachea was infiltrated with additional lidocaine to avoid cough reflex. A circumferential dissection of the stenotic tract or tumor was performed to preserve the recurrent nerves and tracheal vascularization (**Fig. 2**). Then, the stenosis or

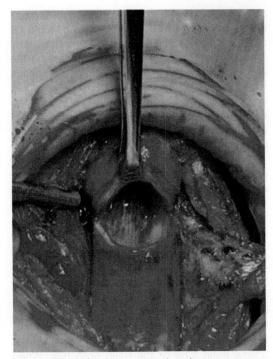

Fig. 1. The trachea was opened under spontaneous ventilation.

tumor was posteriorly dissected from the esophagus.

Stay sutures were placed laterally through the cartilage on each cut edge to align the tracheal ends. The membranous trachea was anastomosed without excessive tension using a 3-0 absorbable running suture, and then the lateral and anterior parts of the anastomosis were completed with interrupted 3-0 absorbable

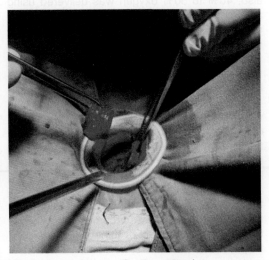

Fig. 2. The trachea tumor was resected.

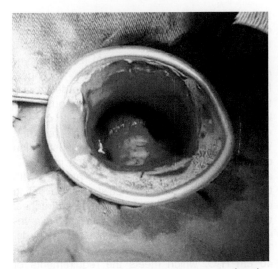

Fig. 3. The end-to-end anastomosis was completed.

sutures (**Fig. 3**). A single cervical drain and a temporary minitracheostomy were placed. Two guardian stitches were placed between the chin and the chest over the manubrium to prevent head and neck extension.

Intrathoracic Trachea Resection and Reconstruction Under Video-Associated Thoracoscopy

The authors have described the technique of intrathoracic trachea resection and reconstruction under VATS and reported a case in 2017.[17] The patient was placed in the lateral decubitus position after being anesthetized. Incisions were made according to the lesion length after administration of local anesthetics at the area. Under thoracoscopy, the azygos vein was separated and stapled with a vascular stapler. After the mediastinal pleura were opened, the vagus nerve was dissected and suspended. Subsequently, the trachea was divided from the level of the suprasternal notch to the carina. After the trachea had been exposed, the operator carried out needle-guided bronchoscopy to reconfirm the extent of tumor margins and then opened the trachea (**Fig. 4**). Reconstruction was initiated after a review of frozen sections confirmed that the margins on both sides were negative.

Reconstruction began from the membranous area of the upper trachea using 3-0 nonabsorbable continuous sutures (**Fig. 5**). Without the endotracheal tube or cross-field ventilation, the operative view was improved considerably and the anastomosis was completed rapidly. After an anastomotic leak and active bleeding had been excluded, 3-0 nonabsorbable continuous sutures

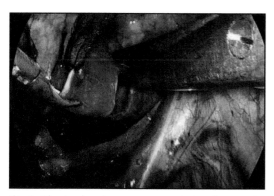

Fig. 4. The trachea tumor was resected under spontaneous ventilation.

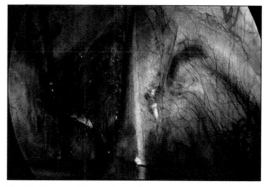

Fig. 6. The end-to-end anastomosis was completed.

were used to enhance the anastomosis. An intrathoracic chest drainage tube was inserted, and the incision was then closed (**Fig. 6**). Finally, 2 prophylactic chin sutures were placed to fix the neck and to reduce extra tension on the anastomosis. To prevent ischemia, the authors suggest the following: (1) the normal trachea should be preserved as long as possible and devascularization should be kept to a minimum; (2) the tissues surrounding the trachea should be protected; and (3) the prophylactic chin sutures preclude the necessity for an extension to improve the local blood supply.

Carinal Resection and Reconstruction

The authors have described the technique of carinal resection and reconstruction and reported a case in 2016.[16] The surgical incisions were selected as follows: (1) observation port: in the sixth intercostal space at anterior axillary line; (2) auxiliary operation port: at posterior line; and (3) main operation port: in the fourth intercostal space between anterior axillary line and midaxillary line. Incision lengths were decided according to tumor length. Local anesthesia with lidocaine was performed before incision creation. After

entering the pleural cavity, the authors blocked the intercostal nerve and the vagus nerve using ropivacaine (0.75%) and lidocaine (2%). The hilar structures were released first, during which the Azygos vein was transected, and the connective tissues at the lower trachea and around the left and right main bronchus were dissociated. During the surgery, the blood supply of the trachea should be carefully protected, and any injury to the vagus nerve should be avoided. Before opening the airway, the surgical field must be kept clean. The right and left main bronchus were transected at the site according to tumor position (**Fig. 7**). Intraoperative frozen-section histopathology was performed to ensure that there was no tumor cell infiltration at the stumps.

During the carinal reconstruction, the lower segment of trachea and the posterior wall of main bronchus were continuously anastomosed using 3-0 nonabsorbable continuous sutures, followed by the anastomosis of the anterior wall (**Fig. 8**). Then, the other main bronchus and the orifice were continuously anastomosed using 3-0 nonabsorbable continuous sutures in the same way. Because there was no tracheal tube,

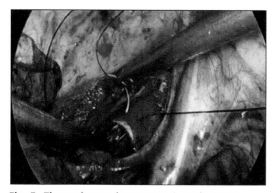

Fig. 5. The end-to-end anastomosis under VATS.

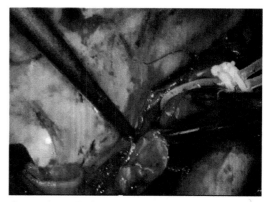

Fig. 7. The carinal tumor was resected under spontaneous ventilation.

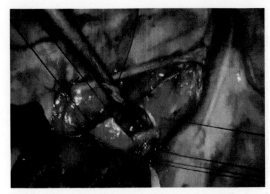

Fig. 8. The carinal reconstruction under VATS.

the surgical field was clearly exposed, making the anastomosis less difficult. An air-leak test using normal saline proved the integrity of the anastomosis (**Fig. 9**). One or 2 chest tubes were placed on the upper and lower pleural cavity after the surgery. The forward head posture was maintained after surgery, with the jaw being fixed with the breast skin using 2 stitches.

COMMENTS

Endotracheal intubation after anesthesia induction and subsequent cross-field ventilation are a widely chosen and standard airway management for tracheal/carinal resection and reconstruction.[4] The safety and applicability to most clinical scenarios have been demonstrated in large patient collectives; it is also the standard care and is accepted by most surgeons. Schieren and colleagues[21] conducted a systematic review that most publications (71.2%) use conventional intubation in their surgical process. Although the number of cases managed with the new technique, like nonintubated spontaneous thoracic surgery, is low, this approach may be beneficial for selected patients.

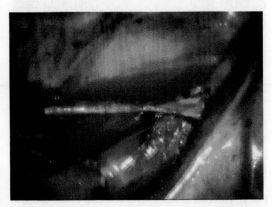

Fig. 9. The carinal reconstruction was completed.

Nonintubated spontaneous thoracic surgery has gained its popularity increasingly in the past decade for the purpose of reducing such adverse events caused by the regimens of general anesthesia.[7] In 1997, Nezu and colleagues[22] initially assessed the feasibility of thoracoscopic wedge resection under spontaneous pneumothorax with local anesthesia, declaring it a safe and beneficial alternative to the conventionally intubated general anesthesia surgery because it provided significantly shorter hospital stays and less invasion. After that, numerous studies have manifested that nonintubated thoracic surgery may be successfully applied to various thoracic conditions,[23] ranging from pneumothorax,[24] malignant pleural effusion,[25] parapneumonic empyema,[26] resection of pulmonary nodules,[27] to tracheal/carinal resection and reconstruction,[16] with the potential benefits including faster postoperative recovery, fewer complications, and shorter hospital stays.

The avoidance of muscle relaxants in nonintubated spontaneous patients may prevent adverse respiratory effects caused by residual muscle block, ranging from diaphragmatic dysfunctions, weakness of upper airway muscles, and airway obstruction to hypoxemia, and thus, accelerates recovery.[20] Jiang and colleagues[28] reported that intubated anesthesia was associated with more postoperative myasthenic crisis than spontaneous patients under thymoma resection, which supported the use of nonintubation for mediastinal tumor surgery. Furthermore, less damage to the trachea, less oxidative response owing to intubation, and better immune function after surgery in the spontaneous group would also contribute to a shorter length of stay after surgery.[10]

From the authors' experience, the indications of such a technique are as follows: (1) neither surgical nor anesthesia contraindications, (2) no severe cardiopulmonary diseases, and (3) less airway secretion. Meanwhile, to ensure the safety and feasibility of the surgical process, some exclusion criteria should be applied: (1) obesity (BMI $\geq$25 kg/m^2), (2) impaired cardiopulmonary function (American Society of Anesthesiologists class 3 or above), (3) respiratory infection, (4) long surgical duration (>5 hours), and (5) difficult airway (Mallampati classification >3). Moreover, to ensure the safety during the procedure, an intubation, cross-field ventilation kit, and mechanical ventilation must be prepared in the case of emergency. Endotracheal intubation or thoracoscopic intubation should be considered in cases with the following conditions: (1) the Spo$_2$ was lower than 90%; (2) continuous carbon dioxide retention, along with the development of respiratory acidosis; and (3) sudden uncontrollable bleeding.

Traditional trachea surgery needs the support of intubation anesthesia 3 times sequentially: (1) initial endotracheal tube before tumor resection, (2) chest (cross-field) intubation in the bronchi after tumor resection, and (3) another oral endotracheal tube in the bronchi after trachea membrane reconstruction. This procedure could be particularly difficult when the stenosis or tumor is severe. Compared with the intubation, nonintubated anesthesia makes the tracheal reconstruction much simpler. Moreover, because of the nature of the blood supply to the trachea, ischemia is a common complication after tracheal surgery; without the inference of intubation, anastomosis become easier and faster, which will decrease the time of ischemia reperfusion for trachea and potentially increase the recovery. Besides, the lack of the tracheal tube facilitated identification and resection of the lesion and then the reconstruction of the trachea, and the spontaneous ventilation that also allowed the opportunity to test the nerves' integrity during the procedure.

Airway tumors and stenoses are rare in thoracic diseases; thus, it is different to conduct a prospective randomized study to confirm the safety and better efficacy of nonintubated anesthesia for tracheal/carinal resection and reconstruction compared with traditional intubation. However, from the evidence of case series and case reports, nonintubated anesthesia is a feasible approach, and it is potentially associated with an easier operation process for surgeons as well as offers better recovery for patients.

ACKNOWLEDGMENTS

All the authors were involved in the conception and design of the study. H. Liang, D. Gonzalez-Rivas, and S. Li contributed to the writing of the article. All the authors critically reviewed and approved the final article.

REFERENCES

1. Handa A, Fujita K, Yamamoto Y, et al. Tracheal tumor. J Pediatr 2016;173. 262–262.e1.
2. Auchincloss HG, Mathisen DJ. Tracheal stenosis-resection and reconstruction. Ann Cardiothorac Surg 2018;7:306–8.
3. Mathisen D. Distal tracheal resection and reconstruction: state of the art and lessons learned. Thorac Surg Clin 2018;28:199–210.
4. Chitilian HV, Bao X, Mathisen DJ, et al. Anesthesia for airway surgery. Thorac Surg Clin 2018;28: 249–55.
5. Kelly GT, Faraj R, Zhang Y, et al. Pulmonary endothelial mechanical sensing and signaling, a story of focal adhesions and integrins in ventilator induced lung injury. Front Physiol 2019;10:511.
6. Marin-Corral J, Dot I, Boguna M, et al. Structural differences in the diaphragm of patients following controlled vs assisted and spontaneous mechanical ventilation. Intensive Care Med 2019;45:488–500.
7. Elkhayat H, Gonzalez-Rivas D. Non-intubated uniportal video-assisted thoracoscopic surgery. J Thorac Dis 2019;11:S220–2.
8. Guo Z, Yin W, Pan H, et al. Video-assisted thoracoscopic surgery segmentectomy by non-intubated or intubated anesthesia: a comparative analysis of short-term outcome. J Thorac Dis 2016;8: 359–68.
9. Guo Z, Yin W, Zhang X, et al. Primary spontaneous pneumothorax: simultaneous treatment by bilateral non-intubated videothoracoscopy. Interact Cardiovasc Thorac Surg 2016;23:196–201.
10. Liu J, Cui F, Pompeo E, et al. The impact of non-intubated versus intubated anaesthesia on early outcomes of video-assisted thoracoscopic anatomical resection in non-small-cell lung cancer: a propensity score matching analysis. Eur J Cardiothorac Surg 2016;50:920–5.
11. Okuda K, Moriyama S, Haneda H, et al. Recent advances in video-assisted transthoracic tracheal resection followed by reconstruction under non-intubated anesthesia with spontaneous breathing. J Thorac Dis 2017;9:2891–4.
12. Atkins JH, Mirza N. Anesthetic considerations and surgical caveats for awake airway surgery. Anesthesiol Clin 2010;28:555–75.
13. Macchiarini P, Rovira I, Ferrarello S. Awake upper airway surgery. Ann Thorac Surg 2010;89:387–90 [discussion: 390–1].
14. Jiang L, Liu J, Gonzalez-Rivas D, et al. Thoracoscopic surgery for tracheal and carinal resection and reconstruction under spontaneous ventilation. J Thorac Cardiovasc Surg 2018;155:2746–54.
15. Shao W, Phan K, Guo X, et al. Non-intubated complete thoracoscopic bronchial sleeve resection for central lung cancer. J Thorac Dis 2014;6:1485–8.
16. Peng G, Cui F, Ang KL, et al. Non-intubated combined with video-assisted thoracoscopic in carinal reconstruction. J Thorac Dis 2016;8:586–93.
17. Guo M, Peng G, Wei B, et al. Uniportal video-assisted thoracoscopic surgery in tracheal tumour under spontaneous ventilation anaesthesia. Eur J Cardiothorac Surg 2017;52:392–4.
18. Caronia FP, Loizzi D, Nicolosi T, et al. Tubeless tracheal resection and reconstruction for management of benign stenosis. Head Neck 2017;39: E114–7.
19. Park SY, Chun HR, Kim MG, et al. Transient Horner's syndrome following thoracic epidural anesthesia for

mastectomy: a prospective observational study. Can J Anaesth 2015;62:252–7.

20. Liu J, Li S, Shen J, et al. Non-intubated resection and reconstruction of trachea for the treatment of a mass in the upper trachea. J Thorac Dis 2016;8:594–9.

21. Schieren M, Bohmer A, Dusse F, et al. New approaches to airway management in tracheal resections–a systematic review and meta-analysis. J Cardiothorac Vasc Anesth 2017;31:1351–8.

22. Nezu K, Kushibe K, Tojo T, et al. Thoracoscopic wedge resection of blebs under local anesthesia with sedation for treatment of a spontaneous pneumothorax. Chest 1997;111:230–5.

23. Mineo TC, Tamburrini A, Perroni G, et al. 1000 cases of tubeless video-assisted thoracic surgery at the Rome Tor Vergata University. Future Oncol 2016;12:13–8.

24. Hwang J, Shin JS, Son JH, et al. Non-intubated thoracoscopic bullectomy under sedation is safe and comfortable in the perioperative period. J Thorac Dis 2018;10:1703–10.

25. Cox SE, Katlic MR. Non-intubated video-assisted thoracic surgery as the modality of choice for treatment of recurrent pleural effusions. Ann Transl Med 2015;3:103.

26. Hsiao CH, Chen KC, Chen JS. Modified single-port non-intubated video-assisted thoracoscopic decortication in high-risk parapneumonic empyema patients. Surg Endosc 2017;31:1719–27.

27. Yang SM, Wang ML, Hung MH, et al. Tubeless uniportal thoracoscopic wedge resection for peripheral lung nodules. Ann Thorac Surg 2017;103(2):462–8.

28. Jiang L, Depypere L, Rocco G, et al. Spontaneous ventilation thoracoscopic thymectomy without muscle relaxant for myasthenia gravis: comparison with "standard" thoracoscopic thymectomy. J Thorac Cardiovasc Surg 2018;155:1882–9.e3.

Nonintubated Tracheal Surgery

Andrey Akopov, MD, PhD*, Mikhail Kovalev, MD, PhD

KEYWORDS

- Benign tracheal stenosis • Tracheal resection • Nonintubated • Supraglottic airway device
- Stenting

KEY POINTS

- The cervical trachea can be resected without endotracheal intubation (nonintubated resection) under jet ventilation performed via a catheter advanced through the supraglottic airway device.
- Supraglottic airway device have several advantages compared with endotracheal tubes in the anesthetic management of patients with benign stenosis in the upper part of the trachea.
- The use of metal stents for temporary airway recanalization, followed by tracheal resection, is an alternative to traditional methods (eg, bouginage or dilatation), which helps avoid the use of an endotracheal tube.
- Preliminary airway stenting and usage of supraglottic airway device makes the formation of tracheal or laryngotracheal anastomosis more convenient compared with traditional endotracheal intubation.

INTRODUCTION

Tracheal resection with direct tracheal or laryngotracheal anastomosis is the best method of radical treatment of benign tracheal stenosis.[1] This approach (especially when stenosis is located in the cervical trachea) is quite simple and, when performed by an experienced surgeon, provides satisfactory immediate and long-term results. Up to 50% of the trachea, whose average total length is 9 to 12 cm, can be safely resected. If a longer part of the trachea needs to be removed, the risk of anastomotic failure and stenosis recurrence increases considerably. That is why numerous surgeons do not consider such resections a feasible option. However, surgery should remain the method of choice for managing the tracheal stenosis that involves less than 50% of the organ length.

Particular attention should be given to lung ventilation during tracheal surgery. Because airway integrity is compromised during surgery, adequate lung ventilation becomes a challenging

issue.[2] Intubation, traditionally used during resections, does not seem to be the best option for several reasons.

This article describes an anesthetic management strategy for resection of the cervical trachea due to benign tracheal strictures. The proposed strategy includes the following steps: (1) insertion of an airway stent in the stenotic area, (2) insertion of a supraglottic airway device (SGAD), and (3) advancing a jet ventilation catheter through the SGAD. Owing to the proposed approach, the tracheal patency and ventilation can be maintained during surgery without using an endotracheal tube (ETT).

CONVENTIONAL METHODS OF ANESTHETIC MANAGEMENT IN TRACHEAL SURGERY

Patient preparation for tracheal surgery starts with a thorough consideration of possible outcomes associated with the condition that required prolonged endotracheal intubation or tracheostomy

Disclosure: The authors have nothing to disclose.
6/8 L/Tolstoy Street, Saint-Petersburg 197022, Russia
* Corresponding author.
E-mail address: akopovand@mail.ru

(eg, brain injury, severe myocardial infarction), which led to the tracheal stenosis.[3] Also, limitations arising from concomitant conditions and their management should be taken into account.[4]

Usually, premedication includes mild sedation (anxiolysis) because most patients are very eager to proceed with the surgery and have their airway patency restored as soon as possible. The choice of anesthesia presents hardly any difficulties. Total intravenous anesthesia is commonly used, which uses a combination of agents that helps avoid opioid-induced respiratory depression and agitation.[5] Different general anesthesia techniques may be used at different stages of the surgery; for example, an inhalation anesthetic while the breathing circuit remains airtight and an intravenous anesthetic once the airways have been opened to the outside. Such muscle relaxants should be used during surgery that provide the possibility of safely reversing neuromuscular block when the surgery is finished. Proper ventilation to ensure adequate oxygenation is probably the most challenging issue to address after the tracheal lumen has been opened.[6] Traditionally, this is achieved by the use of intubation anesthesia. An ETT is usually placed in the trachea itself or passed further, to one of the mainstem bronchi.[7] The tube can be introduced in the caudal part of the trachea through the incisional wound (bypass breathing) to maintain convective ventilation, or it can be inserted in the cranial part of the trachea with a thinner tube (catheter) advanced through it to the resection area to perform intermittent jet ventilation once the airways have been opened. Tracheal resection may also be performed under so-called apneic oxygenation. This refers to a technique that, after the airway has been opened, supplies a constant oxygen flow through a thin catheter inserted in the ETT whose distal end is placed right above the resection area. This technique, however, cannot ensure proper elimination of carbon dioxide. Over the last few years, another method of intraoperative oxygenation, extracorporeal membrane oxygenation, has become increasingly scarce in tracheal surgery. Each of the above-mentioned approaches has its benefits and drawbacks.

BENEFITS AND DRAWBACKS OF ENDOTRACHEAL INTUBATION

The main advantage of intubation is that it helps successfully control the airway until its integrity has been breached. The end of the ETT is positioned beyond the stenotic area. A flexible endoscope can easily be passed through the tube to the distal part of the trachea to perform airway lavage or correct the position of the tube. After the surgeon has entered the tracheal lumen, a sterile armored ETT is introduced through the incisional wound and passed to the distal part of the trachea; then the tube cuff is inflated and the tube is attached to the ventilator. After that, all manipulations in the surgical area are performed around the tube. Abrupt, rough movements of the surgeon or assistant surgeons may disrupt ventilation airflows. The presence of the ETT at the surgical site makes the work of the surgical team rather inconvenient because it complicates separation of the trachea from the surrounding scar tissue and formation of anastomosis. The tube can be removed from the distal part of the trachea during the most complicated steps of the operation; however, ventilation can be disrupted for 1 or 2 minutes only, and oxygen saturation should be constantly monitored during this period (with the saturation value not dropping below 80%). The use of intubation in tracheal stenosis has still other drawbacks.

When intubation is used during surgery for benign stricture of the cervical trachea, the ETT has to be vigorously pushed through the stenotic area. This is the main drawback of intubation because such pushing inevitably traumatizes the tracheal wall in the area of the future anastomosis. Quite often, intubation requires preliminary dilation of the stenotic area with a rigid bougie; this may result in additional damage to the organ, bleeding, or tear of healthy mucosa. Sometimes, most often in high stenosis, the correct placement of the ETT turns out to be a rather complicated task. Also, the pressure of the inflated cuff may lead to impaired blood flow in the tracheal mucosa, which, in its turn, may affect the anastomosis healing. Although the ETT provides the surgeon with the possibility to easily pass instruments to the distal parts of the trachea and bronchi, the size of these instruments is limited by the internal diameter of the tube, which cannot be very wide because it is used in the stenotic trachea. Also, endoscopic examination of vocal cords cannot be performed while the tube is inside the trachea, even though such examination is sometimes necessary during surgery in the cervical trachea and larynx. Also, the removal of the ETT is not an utterly safe procedure when the anastomosis has already been formed because the anastomotic area may be damaged during extubation. Therefore, it is advisable to prevent the most common drawbacks of intubation so that good immediate and long-term results can be achieved after surgery. Despite the above-mentioned disadvantages of the method, an overwhelming number of surgeons accept the use of intubation during tracheal surgery.

JET VENTILATION

Jet ventilation refers to the delivery of high-pressure ventilation gas into the airway through a thin transtracheal catheter. During jet ventilation, the airway is open to the outside, and the respiratory gas is administered under pressure that is considerably higher than usual. There are several types of jet ventilation; for instance, small tidal volumes may be delivered at high frequencies (high-frequency jet ventilation), or greater volumes may be administered at a substantially lower frequency (normal-frequency jet ventilation).[8] The jet ventilation catheter is usually passed into the trachea through the previously inserted ETT. This anesthetic technique provides adequate ventilation of the lower airways and lungs even when the tracheal lumen is open to the outside. Moreover, the diameter of the jet ventilation catheter does not exceed 3 mm, so its presence in the divided trachea (ie, between the cranial and caudal edges of the diastasis after the stenotic part of the trachea has been resected) causes much less interference with required manipulations and allows the surgeon to bring together the tracheal ends and construct an airtight anastomosis. The jet ventilation catheter can be removed from and reintroduced between the ends of the divided airway without any complications because the tracheal lumen can be quite easily accessed via the ETT.

However, jet ventilation requires intubation of the trachea; therefore, all the drawbacks of intubation previously described are also applicable to jet ventilation.

It should be noted that the use of jet ventilation requires an adequate expiratory pathway; that is, adequate gas evacuation from the distant parts of the trachea and lungs. If the air cannot be properly evacuated, the gas can be trapped in the lungs, which may lead to barotrauma; that is, pulmonary overdistention resulting in a unilateral or bilateral pneumothorax. Also, adequate oxygenation may be hard to achieve in patients with decreased lung compliance. Jet ventilation is often associated with hypercapnia.

The device that uses all the advantages of jet ventilation but lacks the drawbacks associated with intubation is an SGAD.[9]

SUPRAGLOTTIC AIRWAY DEVICES

SGADs brands include Laryngeal Mask Airway (LMA) (The Laryngeal Mask Company Ltd., Le Rocher, Victoria Mahe, Republic of Seychelles) and i-gel supraglottic airway (i-gel) (Intersurgical Uab ARNIONI g 60/28-1. LT-16170. PABRADE LITHUANIA), as well as several other devices.

The LMA is a device consisting of an oropharyngeal airway connected to a mask with an inflatable cuff. The air is supplied into the cuff through a non-return valve. The LMA is designed in such a way that it forms an airtight seal around the laryngeal inlet, which ensures a secure airway for both spontaneous respiration and mechanical ventilation during general anesthesia.

The LMA was developed by British anesthesiologist Dr A.I. Brain[10] in 1981. The device concept was based on the idea of maximum control with minimum unwanted effects. The i-gel is an analog of a traditional LMA but is equipped with a soft, gel-like, noninflatable cuff that accurately mirrors the perilaryngeal anatomy. The device is inserted into the hypopharynx. A smooth, atraumatic, thin wall cuff forms an airtight seal and reduces the risk of mucosal damage, allowing a safe access to the larynx. The SGAD does not affect vocal cords, which restore their function under spontaneous breathing.

The SGAD is more easily inserted compared with the ETTs because a less reflexogenic area is involved, local anesthesia may not be used, and the patient may be brought back to consciousness sooner.[11] **Table 1** compares the use of the ETT and the SGAD in tracheal surgery.

Nevertheless, the use of the SGAD in tracheal resection is limited. For example, the device insertion may be complicated in patients with specific anatomic characteristics of the supraglottic area.[12]

The main limitation for the use of the SGAD is associated with complicated lung ventilation in patients with significant stenosis leaving only a very narrow lumen of the airway; in this case, the air volume necessary for adequate ventilation cannot pass the stenotic trachea.

This drawback can be addressed by passing a jet ventilation catheter through the SGAD. This way, the ventilation gas will reach the lower airways. It is not recommended to advance the catheter through the stenotic area, however, because this may increase the risk of pulmonary barotrauma due to improper gas elimination from the trachea and bronchi (improper exhalation).[13] Preliminary dilation of the airway with a bouginage (the disadvantages of this approach are previously described) or a temporary insertion of a tracheal stent can ensure appropriate evacuation of the ventilation gas through the stenotic area.

AIRWAY STENTS IN TRACHEAL STENOSIS

The proposed strategy of the use of the SGAD with the omission of endotracheal intubation can be safely implemented only in those patients

Table 1
Advantages of supraglottic airway devices compared with endotracheal tubes during tracheal resection

Factor	ETT	SGAD
Proper ventilation	Correct placement is nearly impossible in high stenosis	Achieved regardless of the stenosis location
Cough reflex	Elicits	The trachea is not irritated
Local effects in pathologic area	ETT cuff affects the blood flow in the tracheal wall	Does not affect the prognosis for anastomosis healing
Appropriate endoscopic control of vocal cords and tracheobronchial tree	Limits	Allows
Endoluminal passage and control of equipment	Limited by the ETT diameter	Allows
Removal after surgery	Requires thorough control	Safer Reduces the risk of prolonged mechanical ventilation

who have wide enough lumen in the stenotic area to ensure adequate exhalation. Clinical observations indicate that for a stenosis of up to 3 to 4 cm in length the tracheal lumen should be 7 mm or wider. A narrower lumen is associated with a greater risk of barotrauma because of gas trapped in the lower airways; each tidal volume of supplied air increases the pressure in bronchioles and alveoli, which may lead to pneumothorax. Inserting an endoprosthesis in the stenotic area several days before surgery can prevent this complication.

The common recommendation is to avoid long-term use of stents in the trachea if the stenotic area can be resected and it is possible to form anastomosis.[14] This recommendation is made because the presence of an airway stent promotes the growth of granulation tissue and enhances inflammation in the tracheal wall, thus aggravating the stenosis. Airway stents are mostly indicated in those patients in whom single-step radical surgery cannot be performed.[15] It is generally accepted that a silicone stent is a first-choice option in benign stenosis because metal stents, though easier to install, are quickly grown over by scar tissue, often cause pressure ulceration, and are hard to remove from the trachea as few as several weeks after placement.[16,17]

On the other hand, self-expanding metal stents used for a short period of time, just enough to prepare a patient for resection and perform intraoperative anesthesia, are quite convenient and do not demonstrate any of their drawbacks arising during the long-term use.

Preoperative placement of a metal stent in the trachea pursues 2 goals:

- Temporary recanalization of the stenotic airways in patients with respiratory decompensation as an alternative to traditional methods (eg, bouginage) to prepare the patient for a radical tracheal resection
- Prevention of barotrauma during tracheal resection due to the widening of the tracheal lumen, which makes the use of an ETT unnecessary.

The size of the stent is chosen individually. It is not advisable that the stent should cover the stenotic area along its entire length. The stent should be placed in the narrowest part of the trachea so that the proximal and distal ends of the stent do not extend beyond the stenotic area (**Figs. 1** and **2**). Metal stents are easily and safely placed with a flexible bronchoscope with the slightest chance of migration. Accurate positioning of the stent restores adequate ventilation for the period sufficient for patient preparation for surgery and during the operation itself until the trachea is transected below the stenosis. The stent is removed during surgery together with the resected part of the trachea.

Because it is known that extended presence of the stent in the stenotic trachea leads to its overgrowth with scar tissue and, as a result, the stent can hardly be removed, the endoprosthesis should be placed not earlier than 2 weeks before the scheduled date of surgery. Scar tissue will not be able to overgrow the stent during such a short period of time, so it can be removed from the trachea undamaged.

A

B

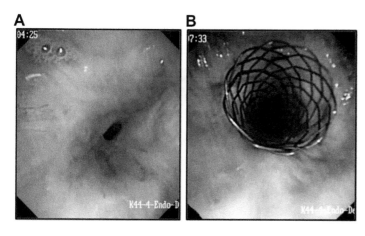

Fig. 1. Preoperative bronchoscopic evaluation of scarred tracheal stenosis. (*A*) Before and (*B*) after stenting.

DESCRIPTION OF THE PROPOSED METHOD
Cooperation Between Surgeon, Anesthesiologist, and Bronchologist

It is of great importance that the surgeon, anesthesiologist, and bronchologist work in close collaboration during tracheal surgery, especially in nonintubated surgery. There exists a risk of inadequate control of ventilation after the airways have been opened. Both the surgeon and the anesthesiologist, each for their own part, should properly control the airway patency and pulmonary ventilation.[18] The bronchologist also has their own part to contribute at each step of the surgery. The surgeon and anesthesiologist should understand well each other's tasks and responsibilities during surgery.

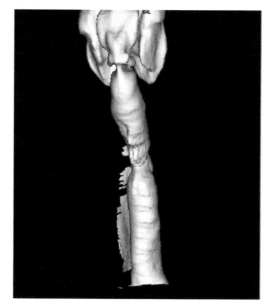

Fig. 2. CT aerogram of a tracheal stenotic segment with an indwelling metallic stent.

It is highly advisable that the surgical team discuss beforehand the plan of surgery, with due consideration given to individual aspects of the clinical case under discussion. The following issues ought to be thought through and assessed carefully: (1) surgical approach, (2) severity of concomitant conditions, (3) the length of the area to be resected, and (4) the distance from the vocal cords to the proximal end of the stenosis.

Such intraoperative complications as incorrect positioning of the ventilation catheter, jamming of the catheter, lower airway obstruction with blood or mucus, or impaired exhalation may develop.[4] Sometimes the catheter previously retracted above the level of the vocal cords cannot be easily returned back into the trachea. This situation can be prevented, however, by putting a thread through the tip of the catheter. This way, the surgeon will be able to pull the thread and return the catheter from the larynx into the trachea. The bronchologist is responsible for the correct positioning of the SGAD and ventilation catheter, sanation of the tracheobronchial tree, and so forth.

The quality of tracheal or laryngotracheal anastomosis is the key to the uncomplicated early and late postoperative course. Using the proposed technique, the surgeon can operate most comfortably, and the anesthesiologist is able to ensure proper ventilation and prevent damage to the anastomosis during the first minutes and hours following surgery.

Procedures Performed by the Anesthesia Care Team

Because some of the preparatory procedures are invasive (eg, insertion of a peripheral arterial line, nasogastric tube, SGAD, flexible laryngotracheobronchoscopy), once in the operating room, the patient is administered mild sedation. The authors consider dexmedetomidine (DEX) to be the safest sedative agent. DEX is an anesthetic agent of choice for tracheal surgery during the entire perioperative period.[6,19,20] The use of DEX helps maintain spontaneous breathing during insertion of airway devices and suppress the cough reflex. Concomitant use of DEX and general anesthetics is associated with additive effects and the possibility of mutual dose reduction. Moreover, DEX has a perioperative opioid-sparing effect, facilitates extubation, suppresses postoperative nausea and vomiting (thus providing additional protection for anastomosis), prevents postoperative agitation and delirium, and is believed to produce antihypoxic effects.[21,22] To achieve moderate sedation (according to the American Society of Anaesthesiologists [ASA]), the optimal combination includes 0.2 to 0.3 mg/kg hour-1 DEX plus 0.5 mg/kg hour-1 propofol and 0.1 mg fentanylum.

The hypopharynx is sprayed with lidocaine 10%. When the nasogastric tube (22F–24 F) has been inserted, the propofol dose is titrated to achieve deep sedation (according to the ASA) for the insertion of the supraglottic airway. We used the i-gel because its noninflatable cuff provides a reduced risk of trauma compared with traditional LMA with an inflatable cuff. The type and size of any supraglottic airway are chosen based on the patient's body weight and the individual anatomy of the oropharynx and hypopharynx. The i-gel device is designed in such a way as to provide free access for endoscopic examination of the laryngeal inlet; it allows for the manipulation of a flexible endoscope, passing the catheter guidewire and the jet ventilation catheter itself to the distal part of the airway, the larynx, and the tracheobronchial tree.[23,24] The authors propose a method that is different from the traditional approach using LMA, in which the jet ventilation catheter is first passed through the larynx and, only after that, the LMA is placed using the catheter as a guide.[13] An adaptor with an airtight seal for an endoscope is connected to the proximal end of the airway. The adaptor, in its turn, is connected to the injector of the high-frequency jet ventilator, which supplies an air–oxygen mixture with varying fractions of inspired oxygen. After the anesthesiologist has performed the laryngoscopy and ascertained that the i-gel is positioned correctly, the catheter guidewire is inserted (**Fig. 3**), and the jet ventilation catheter is passed over the guidewire (**Fig. 4**).

Note that the airway patency ensured by the metal stent preliminary placed in the stenotic trachea helps perform these manipulations without considerable complications. The patient is put under a deeper level of sedation until general anesthesia is achieved; convective, injection, or jet

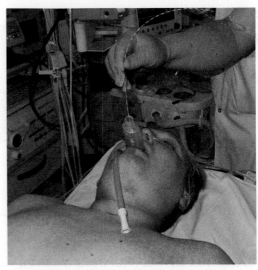

Fig. 3. The guidewire is inserted thorough the I-Gel (Intersurgical Ltd., Wokingham, UK).

ventilation is started. Before switching from spontaneous breathing, the patient is administered a prespecified dose of a muscle relaxant, followed by a maintenance dose under constant neuromuscular blockade monitoring (train-of-four [TOF] monitoring). The ventilator is set to the pressure controlled continuous mandatory ventilation (PC-CMV) mode. The operating pressure for the injection or jet ventilation is preset at 15 mm Hg/kg of body weight, according to general recommendations. The ventilation parameters are adjustable with respect to the arterial blood gas results ($Paco_2$ rate). Jet ventilation with permissive hypercapnia is used once the airways have been

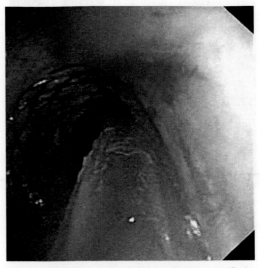

Fig. 4. Bronchoscopic evaluation, the jet ventilation catheter is passed through the tracheal stent.

opened to the outside. The frequency is preset to 100 to 120 per minute, the inspiration time to 40% to 50%, peak airway pressure (Ppeak) limit to less than or equal to 35 mbar, and auto–positive end-expiratory pressure (auto-PEEP) to less than or equal to 6 mbar. The operating pressure is adjusted according to the Pa_{CO_2} values, which are controlled every 30 minutes or as often as required. When the main stage of the operation is finished, and the airtight tracheal anastomosis is formed, the patient is switched to convective CMV. After the anastomosis has been formed, the endoscopic control and sanation of the tracheobronchial tree are performed. Endoscopy aims to (1) examine the larynx for possible postoperative edema (the examination is possible at this stage owing to the supraglottic airway) and (2) visualize the anastomosis from the inside and assess its quality. The anastomosis is tested for leak-tightness by adjusting PEEP so that Ppeak of 30 to 35 mbar can be achieved. If no leakage is detected, the jet ventilation catheter is removed. Concomitantly with continuous infusion of DEX, a maintenance dose of propofol (2–3 mg/ kg × hour^{-1}) is administered; according to our observations, the standard calculated dose of fentanyl used for perioperative analgesia can be reduced. The dosages of the anesthetic agents can be controlled under bispectral index (BIS) monitoring or entropy monitoring. This helps improve patient weaning time. Decurarization (eg, using sugammadex) before removing the i-gel is performed according to a standard protocol when the TOF ratio has returned to at least 90%. The supraglottic airway is usually removed under mild sedation. Once general anesthesia has been reversed, the patient is transferred to the ICU to be followed up until the morning of day 1 after surgery.

Procedures Performed by the Surgical Team

One may not notice any significant differences between procedures performed by an experienced surgeon and his or her assistants during intubated and nonintubated tracheal resection. The surgical team follows a very similar, though somewhat altered, plan of the operation. During nonintubated resection, the surgeon does not waste time on the repositioning of the ETT. The tracheal stent serves as an additional marker for the stenosis location; when the trachea has been separated from the surrounding tissues, the distal resection edge is easily distinguished by palpation. With the metal stent placed inside the trachea, a greater part of the trachea can be spared during resection; the stent itself is

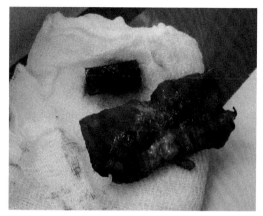

Fig. 5. Resected part of trachea removed during surgery together with a stent.

removed together with the stenotic area (Fig. 5). Once the stenosis has been resected, particular attention is paid to the position of the jet ventilation catheter (Fig. 6). It is the responsibility of an assistant surgeon to fixate the catheter and perform sanation of the distal parts of the tracheobronchial tree.

The posterior wall of the anastomosis is usually formed using a continuous suture (size 3-0 or 4-0 polydioxanone [Ethicon, Inc,Cincinnati, Ohio]), quite often under peripheral oxygen saturation-controlled apnea; the jet ventilation catheter is pulled up so that its end is placed above the proximal edge of the anastomosis. The anterior wall of the anastomosis is formed using an interrupted suture (size 3-0 Vicryl [Ethicon, Inc,Cincinnati, Ohio]). As previously noted, once the formation of the anastomosis has been finished, the surgical team

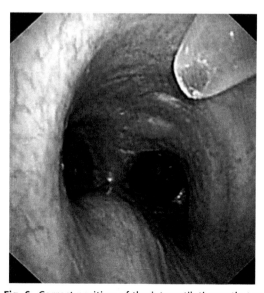

Fig. 6. Correct position of the jet ventilation catheter above the carina.

performs endoscopy. Laryngeal edema is a strong indication for replacing the SGAD with an ETT until layered wound closure and antiedematous therapy are performed.[3] Either the introducer technique or endoscopic support (preferably) is used. Readiness for extubation is assessed in the morning of day 1 after surgery. Continued sedation with DEX prevents the discomfort arising from prolonged endotracheal intubation in patients with restored spontaneous breathing. The wound is closed with a drainage tube placed in the left paratracheal space. After that, 2 thick chin-to-chest sutures are applied in order to prevent hyperextension of the neck during the first days after surgery rather than to maintain the neck in the full flexion. The drainage tube is connected to the negative pressure aspirator (5 mm Hg) and left in the wound until day 1 after surgery. The chin-to-chest sutures are removed on day 7 to 10.

SUMMARY

Tracheal surgery is one of the most technically complicated areas of thoracic surgery. It requires well-coordinated cooperation of the surgeon, anesthesiologist, and bronchologist. It is advisable for each of the specialists to create a safe and comfortable environment for one another. The technique of nonintubated resection of the upper part of the trachea allows the surgeon to work most comfortably and helps the anesthesiologist properly maintain the patient's vital functions in the operating room. The nonintubated surgery using the SGAD can be implemented in combination with previous stenting of the narrowest part of the stenosis; a metal stent is placed in the trachea for a short period of time, just enough to prepare the patient for operation and perform the resection itself. The stent is removed during surgery together with the resected part of the trachea. The observations from the use of the proposed technique in surgical practice indicate that it can be successfully used by specialists who have rich experience in cooperative decision-making in complicated thoracic surgery cases.

REFERENCES

1. Grillo HC. Development of tracheal surgery: a historical review. Part 1: techniques of tracheal surgery. Ann Thorac Surg 2003;75:610–9.
2. Bussières J. Airway management during tracheal resection. In: Deslauriers J, Mehran R, editors. Hand-book of perioperative care in general thoracic surgery. Philadelphia: Elsevier Mosby; 2005. p. 704.
3. Sihag S, Wright CD. Prevention and management of complications following tracheal resection. Thorac Surg Clin 2015;25:499–508.
4. Shamji FM, Deslauriers J. Sharing the airway. The importance of communication between Anesthesiologist and surgeon. Thorac Surg Clin 2018;28:257–61.
5. Chitilian HV, Bao X, Mathisen DJ, et al. Anesthesia for airway surgery. Thorac Surg Clin 2018;28:249–55.
6. Hatipoglu Z, Turktan M, Avci A. The anesthesia of trachea and bronchus surgery. J Thorac Dis 2016;8:3442–51.
7. Hobai IA, Chhangani SV, Alfille PH. anesthesia for tracheal resection and reconstruction. Anesthesiol Clin 2012;30:709–30.
8. Pinsonneault C, Fortier J, Donati F. Tracheal resection and reconstruction. Can J Anaesth 1999;46:439–55.
9. Biro P, Hegi TR, Weder W, et al. Laryngeal mask airway and high-frequency jet ventilation for the resection of a high-grade upper tracheal stenosis. J Clin Anesth 2001;13:141–3.
10. Brain AI. The laryngeal mask airway: a new concept in airway management. Br J Anaesth 1983;55:801–4.
11. Krecmerova M, Schutzner J, Michalek P, et al. Laryngeal mask for airway management in open tracheal surgery-a retrospective analysis of 54 cases. J Thorac Dis 2018;10:2567–72.
12. Zardo P, Kreft T, Hachenberg T. Airway management via laryngeal mask in laryngotracheal resection. Thorac Cardiovasc Surg Rep 2016;5:1–3.
13. Wiedemann K, Männle C. Anesthesia and gas exchange in tracheal surgery. Thorac Surg Clin 2014;24:13–25.
14. Walters DM, Wood DE. Operative endoscopy of the airway. J Thorac Dis 2016;8S:130–9.
15. Colt H, Murgu S. Post intubation tracheal stenosis. the resection itself. The stent is removed during. In: Colt H, Murgu S, editors. Bronchoscopy and central airway disorders. Philadelphia: Elsevier Saunders; 2012. p. 95–103.
16. Ayub A, Al-Ayoubi AM, Bhora FY. Stents for airway strictures: selection and results. J Thorac Dis 2017;9S:116–21.
17. Semaan R, Yarmus L. Rigid bronchoscopy and silicone stents in the management of central airway obstruction. J Thorac Dis 2015;7S:352–62.
18. Lingard L, Garwood S, Poenaru D. Tensions influencing operating room team function: does institutional context make a difference. Med Educ 2004;38:691–9.
19. Ramsay MAE, Saha D, Hebeler RF. Tracheal resection in the morbidly obese patient: the role of dexmedetomidine. J Clin Anesth 2006;18:452–4.
20. Kashii T, Nabatame M, Okura N, et al. Successful use of the i-gel and dexmedetomidine for tracheal

resection and construction surgery in a patient with severe tracheal stenosis. Masui 2016;65:366–9.

21. Sharma S, Jain P. Dexmedetomidine and anesthesia. Int J Clin Pharm 2013;24:223–5.

22. Mantz J, Josserand J, Hamada Ş. Dexmedetomidine: new insights. Eur J Anaesthesiol 2011;28:3–6.

23. Arévalo-Ludeña J, Arcas-Bellas JJ, Alvarez-Rementería R, et al. Fiberoptic-guided intubation after insertion of the i-gel airway device in spontaneously breathing patients with difficult airway predicted: a prospective observational study. J Clin Anaesth 2016;35:287–92.

24. Polat R, Aydin GB, Ergil J, et al. Comparison of the i-gel™ and the Laryngeal Mask Airway Classic™ in terms of clinical performance. Rev Bras Anestesiol 2015;65:343–8.

Management of Intraoperative Crisis During Nonintubated Thoracic Surgery

Jose Navarro-Martínez, MD, EDAIC[a],*, Maria Galiana-Ivars, MD[a],
María Jesús Rivera-Cogollos, MD[a], Carlos Gálvez, MD, PhD[b],
Sergio Bolufer Nadal, MD, PhD[b], Marta Ortega Lamaignère[c],
Elena Díez Mazo[c]

KEYWORDS

• Anesthesia • Thoracic surgery • Nonintubated • Crisis • Management

KEY POINTS

- The benefits of nontubated video-assited thoracoscopic surgery are based on the less invasiveness and earlier recovery. But nevertheless, intraoperative complicactions are possible.
- Correct prevention and management of these potentially critical situations are vital, and the principles of crisis resource management must be followed.
- Crisis resource management must include clinical simulation as a tool to generate different scenarios to improve teamwork.
- Simulation-based crisis resource management training programs for a specific surgery can contribute to reduce frequency and effect of these critical situations.

INTRODUCTION

In recent years, different nonintubated video-assisted thoracoscopic surgery (NIVATS) programs[1,2] with different degrees of complexity[3,4] have been developed, based on less invasiveness and early recovery,[5–7] compared with standard surgery.[8,9] The theoretic benefits are obvious: avoid orotracheal intubation, the adverse effects of using double-lumen tubes, open pneumothorax with better lung collapse, and caudal movement of the diaphragm. There is also a less immunologic and inflammatory impact[10] and even in morbidity and hospital stay.[11,12] Potential risks include hypoxemia, hypercapnia, cough, and severe bleeding. These complications can evolve into a critical situation in which trained personnel is essential.[8,9]

Intraoperative surgical emergencies are included in the high acuity (it assesses the severity of an event and the impact on the patient) and low occurrence (it assess the occurring frequency).[13] This combination puts the patient in a situation in which medical errors can occur more commonly. Although these errors are ubiquitous and unavoidable, one must try to establish the knowledge, skills, and attitudes necessary to achieve proper teamwork and systematically guide the management of a critical event. This strategy would probably reduce the incidence of errors[14] and improve decision making.

Disclosure Statement: The authors have nothing to disclose.
[a] Anesthesiology Department and Surgical Critical Care Unit, Hospital General Universitario de Alicante, C/Pintor Baeza no. 12, Alicante 03010, Spain; [b] Thoracic Surgery Department, Hospital General Universitario de Alicante, C/Pintor Baeza no. 12, Alicante 03010, Spain; [c] Hospital General Universitario de Alicante, C/Pintor Baeza no. 12, Alicante 03010, Spain
* Corresponding author.
E-mail address: jnavarro.martinez@gmail.com

Thorac Surg Clin 30 (2020) 101–110
https://doi.org/10.1016/j.thorsurg.2019.08.009
1547-4127/20/© 2019 Elsevier Inc. All rights reserved.

A strategy for handling these situations comes from the application of the principles of crisis resource management (CRM). CRM tries to develop all the nontechnical skills[15,16] needed in a critical situation, but not only that, it also includes all the tools necessary to prevent it. Can the risks be reduced with an adequate training plan? That is what this article is going to try to answer.

CRISIS RESOURCE MANAGEMENT KEY ELEMENTS APPLIED TO NONINTUBATED VIDEO-ASSISTED THORACOSCOPIC SURGERY

Managing critical events during surgery is one of the most difficult and important tasks required of the surgical team. It was Professor Gaba,[4,5] more than 20 years ago, who introduced the concept of CRM. CRM refers to the set of nontechnical skills[15] required for effective teamwork in a crisis situation, whereby patient safety during surgery is the main objective. The CRM concept was originally developed in the aviation domain. It was initially called "cabin resource management" and later "crew resource management," because of the importance of the group's reaction in a crisis by simulating different scenarios. The key elements of CRM are listed in **Table 1**.

Know the Environment and Available Resources

One of the key elements is to try to prevent the complication from happening. For that reason, knowing your environment and all the available resources is essential. This first set of CRM actions can be called "*before the crisis happens.*" The

available resources can be classified as human (one's own knowledge/skills and the others around him or her), materials, cognitive aids, and other external resources. The human performance resources are not constant throughout the day, because they are affected by fatigue, need of sleep, emotional disturbances, health problems, lack of experience, welfare pressure, and lack of knowledge. From these circumstances, the dangerous attitudes of oneself or one's environment are especially important, examples such as antiauthority, "Don't tell me what to do!"; impulsivity, "Do something quickly"; invulnerability, "That would never happen to me"; macho, "You'll see how I operate it"; resignation, "There's nothing we can do." For these attitudes, antidotes must be found, and, in some cases, a psychologist may even have to be consulted. A second important aspect is the pressure to which the surgical staff is subjected. To control this, multidisciplinary protocols must be approved by all parties involved, in which the day-to-day surgery adapts based on the needs of patients (safety) and not the numbers to be met. Along with that, it is essential to check the correct functioning of the available material resources before starting (how each element works as well as the most frequent faults), making sure that the emergency equipment is immediately available. Other external resources include "who" can be asked for help in an emergency and "where" the things are that are needed.

The NIVATS team must know their own limitations, try to improve them, and have previous experience. To define experienced team, the following criteria are used: surgeons,

---

Table 1
Crisis resource management key elements and nonintubated video-assisted thoracoscopic surgery application

CRM Key Elements	NIVATS Application
1. Know the environment and available resources	• Expert team (>50 VATS cases)
2. Anticipation and plan	• Anesthesiologist trained in the lateral position
3. Call for help soon	• First case of the day
4. Exercise leadership and "followship"	• Emergency table prepared
5. Distribute workload	• Specific informed consent signed by the patient
6. Mobilize all available resources	• At the beginning of the NIVATS program, 2 anesthesiologists in the operation room
7. Communicate effectively	• In case of surgical crisis (bleeding), one of the nurses helps the surgeon, if it is medical (hypoxemia), the nurse helps the anesthesiologist
8. Use all available information	
9. Prevent and manage fixation errors	
10. Double and cross-check	• Specific cognitive aids developed for NIVATS (anestCRITIC)
11. Use cognitive aids	
12. Reevaluate repeatedly	• Use high-fidelity simulators to train: hypoxemia (lateral intubation), severe bleeding (reconversion to thoracotomy), and cardiac arrest in the lateral position
13. Good teamwork	
14. Focus attention wisely	
15. Set priorities dynamically	

anesthesiologists and nurses must have done more than 50 conventional VATS and overcome the learning curve along with experience in difficult cases of large pulmonary resections (large and central tumors, bronchoangioplasties, tumors with invasion of neighboring structures). In addition, they should have faced complications, such as moderate or severe bleeding through VATS. A unique issue is that the anesthesiologist must be trained in the lateral intubation. The authors discuss it in more detail in later discussion. The NIVATS patient, at the beginning of the program, should be scheduled as the first case of the day. The surgical equipment the authors use is the standard VATS. What is different is that they have prepared what they call the "emergency table" (**Box 1**). It is essential that everything is reviewed and prepared.

Box 1
Checklist in nonintubated video-assisted thoracoscopic surgery

Before surgery

- Consent to anesthesia and specific surgery for this procedure
- World Health Organization safety list
- Two anesthesiologists present

Emergency table

Anesthesia

- Facial mask of the size adapted to the patient
- Guedel cannula
- Laryngoscope with 2 blade sizes
- Videolaryngoscope (in the authors' case, the double lumen tube Airtraq)
- Two sizes of double lumen tube (35–37F) orotracheal tubes
- Two sizes of single tracheal tubes (7–7.5 mm)
- Endobronchial blocker (in the authors' case, Uniblocker)
- Frova Guide
- Fibrobronchoscope ready to use (3.7 mm)
- Drugs for the induction of a general anesthetic (propofol + fentanyl + rocuronium)
- Drugs for reversal of muscle relaxant (Sugammadex)

On the instrumentalist table, there will be the following:

- Thoracic drainage (24F)
- Drainage system with water seal, ready to use

Anticipation and Plan

In order to try to avoid patient-related problems, a strict inclusion protocol is applied (included in a checklist). The surgeon and anesthesiologist explain the advantages and disadvantages of NIVATS to the patient, and a specific informed consent is signed. In case of doubt, the patient is excluded. Anticipation helps to avoid surprises because during a crisis surprises are not welcome. Planning ahead eliminates much of the stress in those times of great upheaval. One must to try to wait for the unexpected, and as a pilot would say, "always fly in front of our plane."

Call for Help Soon

Asking for help early is not a sign of lack of self-confidence but demonstrates your respect and sense of responsibility for your patient's safety. Heroes are dangerous. We need to know what kind of help is needed: muscle, transportation, general technical skill, knowledge, or just someone trustworthy. At the beginning of the NIVATS program, the authors had 2 anesthesiologists in the theater, and after gaining experience, at least 1 expert colleague is located in the surgical area. Calling for help is very important to avoid fixing errors in the event of a crisis.

Exercise Leadership and Followers

The first objective is to define the role and functions of the *team*,[17] knowing when to be a leader (leadership) and when to be a follower ("followship"). The leader has to communicate effectively, without raising his voice, indicating orders or needs in the clearest and most precise way possible, avoiding making statements on the air, asking for the confirmation message when something or someone is asked for. The follower must listen to what the leader says and do what is needed always with an open mind to help and convey their concerns to the leader. The focus must be *what* is right and not *who is* right. In case of a surgical emergency (severe bleeding), with the patient stable, the leader is the surgeon. If it is a medical emergency (hypoxemia), the anesthesiologist takes control of the situation and should stop the surgery if deemed necessary. Knowing the type of emergency is important for allocating other human resources (nursing). At the beginning of an NIVATS, the authors have 3 nurses in the operating room. In case of emergency, 1 nurse assists the surgeon, and the other assists the anesthesiologist. In the authors' hospital, they do not have specific anesthesia nurses, which would be ideal.

Distribute the Workload

One of the main tasks of the leader is to distribute the workload. Someone has to define the tasks, check that they are carried out correctly, and check that everything is working properly. If possible, the leader should be freed from other tasks to observe, gather information, and delegate. Team members should actively seek out all those tasks that need to be done. It is not a good team in which its leader has to direct each of its actions.

Mobilize All Available Resources

In order to handle a problem, one should think of everyone and everything that could help to handle the problem. That includes people and technology. As far as the human aspect is concerned, their knowledge and skills as well as knowing their strengths and weaknesses are their most important resources. The resources are there to be used. After a crisis, one often realizes that there were precious resources available that should have been mobilized. They can be human or monitoring and equipment.

Communicate Effectively

Communication is the key in crisis situations. Communication ensures that everyone knows what is going on, what needs to be done, and what is already done, which sometimes is hard. The fact of saying something can be considered a communication if the message is received. Meaning does not mean "to say," saying does not mean "to hear," hearing does not mean "to understand," and understanding does not mean "to do."

Use All Available Information

Medicine is complex because information must be integrated from many different sources. Each piece of information can help one better understand the patient's condition to arrive at a correct diagnosis. Complete the scheme by correlating all the different sources: clinical impression, information from relatives (eg, drug abuse or coexisting diseases), and above all, watch for changes in vital signs.

Prevent and Manage Fixation Errors

The next point to develop is the so-called fixing errors. This type of error is very common in dynamic settings and creates a persistent inability to review

a diagnosis or plan even though the available evidence suggests that review of the diagnosis or plan is necessary. The 3 most common are the following situations: "It is this and only this," we have not taken into account an alternative diagnosis; "Everything but this," neglecting a single diagnosis; "Everything is fine," they do not recognize the need to act in emergency mode. One must try to avoid these errors by checking and rechecking from the outset all the actions that are carried out, even if it is thought that it has been done correctly. Crisis situations are dynamic: what is right now may be wrong the next minute. Fixation errors are errors of the mental model one has of both the patient and the situation. They are therefore difficult to grasp and are presented in a variety of ways. Knowing the enemy helps to answer him. Always rule out the worst-case scenario.

Double and Cross-Check

Cross-checking means correlating data from different sources. Is the artifact seen in the electrocardiogram also seen in the pulse oximeter wave? Memory sometimes deceives and always tries to make things fit together in a logical way. It might not be an artifact. Double-checking is about making sure that what you remember you saw is what you actually saw. As has been said before, sometimes the mind deceives us and you think you did something, but you may not have done it, simply because you thought of doing it but you did not do it. You may have thought of suspending a perfusion, but it turns out that you left it completely open. Check all devices to make sure they are the way you want them to be.

Use Cognitive Aids

It is recommended to use cognitive aids.[18,19] There are different types of cognitive aids (checklist vs lineal vs branched algorithms), but they all have similar functions. The great strength of humans (but also their great weakness) lies in the fact that they tend to take shortcuts, do not think systematically, and are flexible. What, in general, is a help, will cause mistakes when things have to be done in a clear order and without losing any element. That is why humans design cars and robots and make them by following the same pattern over and over again. Using checklists, which are common in other fields, can help one not to forget important steps in diagnosis or treatment. If machines are better than humans in math, why not let them be? Calculating doses using a calculator leads to fewer errors than doing so using one's head. Searching for doses or other information demonstrates responsibility and not lack of knowledge. Never feel bad about looking for something, even if you knew it before and do not remember it anymore. Keep important information in a safe place. Do not be a hero; be responsible. It could be a life or death decision!

A checklist described in **Box 1** is used, where all items must be marked for an NIVATS. Along with this it should be available a cognitive aid either on paper or in an electronic version[20] (anestCRITIC, available in iTunes and Google Play).

Reevaluate Repeatedly

Medicine is dynamic. What is right now may not be right in the next minute. Each piece of information can be important and can change the situation. Although some parameters may change slowly over time, subtle changes can be difficult to perceive. Do not hesitate to follow a dynamic situation by making decisions dynamically (do not go on with the decisions you made if the situation changes).

Good Teamwork

Not all teamwork is good, and getting good teamwork is difficult. The coordination of a team begins before it is assembled. If all members know the work to be done and their roles within this work, coordination is easier. To this end, several meetings have been held before the start of the project (**Fig. 1**), including clinical simulations using high-fidelity simulators. Respect team members and

their "weaknesses." The "players" of the team must be attentive to the needs of the people next to them. Work hand in hand.

Focus Attention Wisely

Because human's attention is very limited, and humans are not good at doing several things at once, you will find yourself several times in the situation of having to share your attention. Two principles may be useful to you. First, it is reasonable to develop sequences or rhythms; the ABC sequence (Airway, Breathing, Circulation) is based on this principle. If you can maintain this sequence, you are less likely to lose important details. The second principle is to alternate between focusing on the details and focusing on the whole picture. Whenever you need to focus on 1 detail (eg, difficult intubation), try to force yourself to go back to the full picture and reevaluate the patient's overall situation. Try not to be distracted; interrupt long processes and check the patient's condition.

Set Priorities Dynamically

Dynamic situations need dynamic measures. Do not stick to your decisions, because they are often based on incomplete and not entirely true information. What was right before may not be right now and vice versa. Having a solution does not mean having the best solution. However, there is 1 priority that is absolute and that is to keep the patient's vital signs stable at all times. Even if you do not

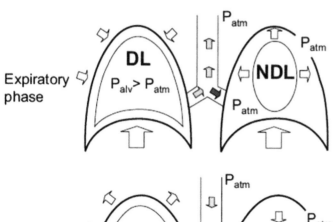

Fig. 1. Distribution of ventilation in a lateral decubitus patient with a surgical pneumothorax. During exhalation, the air comes out (*blue arrows*) from the DL. Part of that air (*red arrow*) enters the NDL as the P_{alv} equals the P_{atm}. During inspiration, part of the NDL air enters the DL contributing to hypoventilation. P_{alv}, alveolar pressure; P_{atm}, atmospheric pressure; PD, dependent lung; PND, nondependent lung.

know what is happening to the patient, take care of your constants and do not get lost in mental thoughts while the patient stops breathing.

SPECIFIC CLINICAL AND CRITICAL SITUATIONS

In order to understand which situations we may find ourselves in, we first need to know the physiopathology of surgical pneumothorax in NIVATS.[21,22] Nondependent lung collapse begins once atmospheric pressure contacts the pleural cavity and will be proportional to the opening in the chest. If the patient is in the lateral position, with spontaneous breathing and the induced pneumothorax, 2 things must be considered: first, displacement of the mediastinum toward the dependent lung, owing to the loss of negative pressure of the nondependent lung; second, paradoxic breathing (see **Fig. 1**); during inspiration, the nondependent lung collapses and expands during exhalation. Both changes decrease the efficiency of spontaneous ventilation with reinspiration of exhaled gases. Respiratory function may be aggravated by blockage of intercostal muscles by regional anesthesia and excess sedation required for the patient.

Respiratory Acidosis

Permissive hypercapnia is very common in NIVATS and is directly dependent on the duration of the surgery and the sedation level. It could be a big issue if it is not controlled properly. For that reason, the authors monitor $Paco_2$ through the radial artery and sequential blood gas analysis. In case of severe hypercapnia, the authors assist the patient with a facial mask. The use of high-flow ventilation (using intermediate flows) might potentially show benefit in carbon dioxide washout without recruiting the nondependent lung,[23] but this should be studied in prospective randomized clinical trials. Some teams defend the use of a laryngeal mask to ensure patency of the airway, to keep spontaneous breathing while available for mechanical ventilation.[24]

Hypoxemia

The degree of hypoxemia varies greatly depending on the type of patient. As can be see, in thoracic patients, the drop-in oxygen saturation is usually greater in "healthy" patients or in those who do not have preexisting lung problems. During surgery, the goal is to maintain oxygen saturation greater than 95%. This goal is usually achieved by administering oxygen through a standard facial mask. Again, in case of a major hypoxemia, the

authors first use a high-flow ventilation of oxygen with the lowest possible flow of usually 20 to 30 L/min. If the patient persists in being hypoxemic, the next step is intubation. The use of noninvasive facial ventilation has not been studied.

Dyspnea

At the beginning of the NIVATS program, a more superficial level of sedation was used, and it was explained to the patient that at the beginning of the procedure, when the pneumothorax was done, he or she could notice "shortness of breath." Currently, because deeper levels are used, the patient does not usually experience this sensation. In the case of being at the beginning of an NIVATS program, it is recommended to explain to the patient the possibility of feeling dyspnea.

Cough

One of the most common problems during NIVATS is the patient's cough. Cough receptors are found mainly in the posterior wall of the trachea, pharynx, and bronchial mucosa. All coughs are mediated by the vagus nerve. The predominance of vagal tone after sympathetic blockage by the use of an epidural catheter could theoretically increase bronchial tone and reactivity.

There are several ways to block this cough reflex,[25] but none of them suppresses it 100% and without risk: The first option is to administer 1 to 2 mg/kg lidocaine intravenously and then a continuous perfusion, but there is a risk of toxicity. The second way is to use the 2% to 4% aerosol inhalation of lidocaine in a high flow of oxygen for about 30 minutes before surgery. The third option is to make an intrathoracic vagal block with 2 mL bupivacaine at 0.25% adjacent to the vagus nerve under direct thoracoscopic vision at the level of the azygos vein on the right side, and just below the aortopulmonary window on the left side. This option has a variant that consists of spraying 0.25% bupivacaine in the visceral pleura and posterior mediastinal pleura following the vagus nerve. Finally, block the ipsilateral stellate ganglion with 10 mL of 0.25% bupivacaine. Despite everything, there are patients in whom cough control is not adequate.

Massive Hemorrhage

In the authors' protocol, the patient has 2 large-caliber short peripheral venous catheters on the contralateral side of the surgery. They do not use central venous lines. In case of massive hemorrhage, they use the same protocol as in any other patient, including tracheal intubation.

CONVERSION CRITERIA

The criteria for conversion to multiportal surgery, thoracotomy, and/or general anesthesia are defined in **Box 2**. The management of 1 situation or another will vary depending on the reason for a medical or surgical reconversion. While in the medical crisis, the authors induce general anesthesia, intubation of the patient, and placement of thoracic drainage through the incision and connection to an aspiration system for pulmonary reexpansion. In the surgical crisis (bleeding), they have less time to react, and the anesthesiologist will try not to ventilate the patient until the double lumen tube (or blocker) is placed correctly (checked by bronchofibroscope). It is done in this manner because in the authors' center, all cases, initially, are performed with a single port of access, so if that lung is ventilated, the emergency solution would be more difficult.

Box 2
Medical and surgical criteria for conversion to thoracotomy and general anesthesia

Medical criteria

- Respiratory acidosis with pH <7.1, with tachypnea (>30 rpm)
- Hypoxemia (Po_2 <60 mm Hg), no improvement despite high oxygenation flow or noninvasive ventilation
- Cough continues without improvement despite sprayed lidocaine or vagal blockage
- Anxiety attack without improvement with sedation

Surgical criteria

Reasons for converting to multiportal VATS

- Extensive adhesions of the lung to the chest wall on more than 50% of its surface in a spontaneously breathing patient
- Large central and anterior tumors that make it difficult to manipulate hilar structures through the single incision
- Inadequate collapsed lung
- Bronchoplasties
- Mild bleeding (small branches of the pulmonary artery and vein, bronchial arteries)

Reasons for conversion to an open thoracotomy

- Severe bleeding requiring more important maneuvers (pulmonary artery clamp, primary suture, reconstruction)
- No palpation of nodules

AIRWAY MANAGEMENT IN NONINTUBATED VIDEO-ASSISTED THORACOSCOPIC SURGERY

NIVATS airway management has also evolved a great deal in a very short time. Two different situations can be found: routine and emergency management. In routine management, the situation has gone from having patients with superficial sedation to having them with deep sedation. This evolution has increased the resultant problems from respiratory depression (hypercapnia and hypoxemia). To prevent problems, the authors have several devices they can use: (a) oropharyngeal cannula (Mayo or Guedel): their use avoids airway obstruction when sedation is deep. (b) Laryngeal masks: their use has increased because, like the first ones, they prevent airway obstruction (if they are well placed), allows the patient to ventilate spontaneously, and improves oxygenation. In return, problems may arise related to the malposition of these during the procedure, which would force the attempt of repositioning. It is advisable to check their placement with a fiberscope. In case of complications, the authors can use it (or the Frova guide) to secure the airway with an orotracheal tube. (c) Simple orotracheal tubes: use of simple orotracheal tubes could also be another option because the use would assure the airway, being able to also maintain the patient spontaneously. Above all, it would allow one to quickly put in a blocker. The problem would be that it would increase resistance to airflow, increasing respiratory work as well.

An important and differential issue of NIVATS is the need for lateral intubation training in the case of an emergency. The residency programs do not include this type of technique, so before the authors start doing NIVATS, they must perform it on scheduled patients. Lateral intubation, in the authors' experience, has several peculiarities. The first thing to be stressed on this point is that this is not technically more difficult than doing it in the supine position. Second, positioning the patient in the lateral position before the anesthesia is induced is very useful for the whole team. The patient can be positioned as comfortably as possible (preventing iatrogenic injuries by the stretching of the brachial plexus). The surgeon can achieve the best surgical approach without injury. The anesthesiologist can intubate without increasing the risk. The whole team benefits from not having to put the patient "at weight." How is the right way to do it? As shown in **Fig. 2**, the head should be in a neutral position, with a pair of pillows and an occipital support to prevent the head from

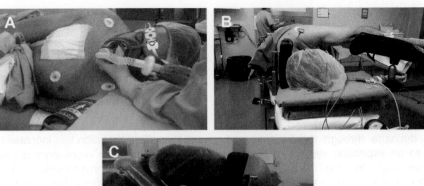

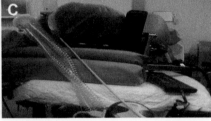

Fig. 2. (*A–C*) Correct placement of the patient in the lateral position. Neutral position of the head with support in the occipital zone. Lateralization of the table toward the opposite side of the intubation.

going backwards during laryngoscopy (simulating the sniffing position).

Ventilation is easier than in the supine position. This position is the safety position to prevent pulmonary aspiration, and hypopharyngeal structures do not tend to obstruct the airway as in supine decubitus. Correct manual ventilation is normally achieved without the need for oropharyngeal cannulas. In theory, intubations in the right lateral position could be somewhat more difficult when it comes to directing the tube (because of the fall of the tongue, which makes it difficult to insert the laryngoscope blade). This difficulty is greatly reduced by rotating the table in the opposite direction. The latter is important because anesthesiologist may have a tendency to turn the head (and not the table) and that can make intubation difficult. Another option would be, directly, to intubate the patient with the videolaryngoscope, with which the authors have more experience. In all situations requiring intubation (whatever device is used), it is advisable to place a Frova guide (removing the metal guide from the double lumen tube, if it is going to be used) to facilitate the direction of the tube and the possibility of being able to oxygenate through its channel.

CLINICAL TRAINING AND SIMULATION

An important aspect, and because of the potential risk of complications, it is advisable to establish a program of NIVATS from minor to major complexity[1] to avoid complications and really objectify a benefit for the patient. This program must go hand-in-hand with a change in the

form of training to which they are subjected, from residents to the recertifications of the most experienced people,[26–28] which include aspects related to assessment by competencies. Clinical simulation should be included in the competency-based assessment.

Last but not least, training is necessary in crisis situations. The use of clinical simulation offers the opportunity to train all the potentially critical elements (**Fig. 3**) surrounding the NIVATS in an objective and repetitive manner.[1] The authors use high-fidelity simulators to train 3 controlled scenarios: hypoxemia and the need of lateral intubation, severe bleeding, and cardiac arrest in the lateral position. Through the use of a specific thoracic cognitive aid (anestCRITIC app in GooglePlay and iTunes), the authors do a judicious debriefing in a constructive manner (**Fig. 4**). The ultimate goal can be achieved: better care and safety for their patients.[29]

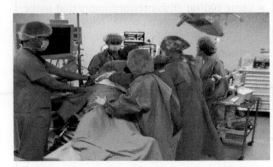

Fig. 3. Simulation of cardiac arrest in the lateral position during thoracic surgery in Hospital General Universitario de Alicante.

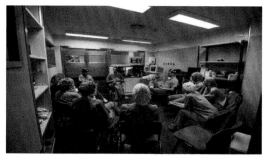

Fig. 4. Debriefing following in situ simulation in the operating room of the Hospital General Universitario de Alicante.

SUMMARY

Medical and surgical emergencies during an NIVATS must follow the principles of CRM. Knowing the resources available, anticipating, planning, and using cognitive aids are the basis for minimizing the risk of complications. Even if we do it perfectly, the crisis happens; that is why it is fundamental to ask for help on time, to know when to lead and when to follow, to distribute the workload, to mobilize all available resources, to communicate effectively, to prevent and manage fixing errors, to check and retest, to use cognitive aids, to reevaluate repeatedly, to work in a team, to focus attention skillfully, and to establish priorities in a dynamic way. Simulation training is a useful tool for the implementation of all of these concepts, without forgetting the most important concept, that the whole team has to be involved. The aim is to improve patient safety and reduce errors to a minimum.

REFERENCES

1. Caviezel C, Schuepbach R, Grande B, et al. Establishing a non-intubated thoracoscopic surgery programme for bilateral uniportal sympathectomy. Swiss Med Wkly 2019;149:w20064.
2. Moon Y, AlGhamdi ZM, Jeon J, et al. Non-intubated thoracoscopic surgery: initial experience at a single center. J Thorac Dis 2018;10:3490–8.
3. Zuin A, Mammana M, Rea F. Non-intubated tracheal surgery: is it worthwhile? J Thorac Dis 2017;9:3663–6.
4. Okuda K, Nakanishi R. The non-intubated anesthesia for airway surgery. J Thorac Dis 2016;8:3414–9.
5. Ali JM, Volpi S, Kaul P, et al. Does the "non-intubated" anaesthetic technique offer any advantage for patients undergoing pulmonary lobectomy? Interact Cardiovasc Thorac Surg 2019;28:555–8.
6. Lirio F, Galvez C, Bolufer S, et al. Tubeless major pulmonary resections. J Thorac Dis 2018;10:S2664–70.
7. Liu J, Cui F, Pompeo E, et al. The impact of non-intubated versus intubated anaesthesia on early outcomes of video-assisted thoracoscopic anatomical resection in non-small-cell lung cancer: a propensity score matching analysis. Eur J Cardio Thorac Surg 2016;50:920–5.
8. Wang M-L, Galvez C, Chen J-S, et al. Non-intubated single-incision video-assisted thoracic surgery: a two-center cohort of 188 patients. J Thorac Dis 2017;9:2587–98.
9. AlGhamdi ZM, Lynhiavu L, Moon YK, et al. Comparison of non-intubated versus intubated video-assisted thoracoscopic lobectomy for lung cancer. J Thorac Dis 2018;10:4236–43.
10. Mineo TC, Sellitri F, Vanni G, et al. Immunological and inflammatory impact of non-intubated lung metastasectomy. Int J Mol Sci 2017;18:1466.
11. Tacconi F, Pompeo E. Non-intubated video-assisted thoracic surgery: where does evidence stand? J Thorac Dis 2016;8:S364–75.
12. Navarro-Martínez J, Gálvez C, Rivera-Cogollos MJ, et al. Intraoperative crisis resource management during a non-intubated video-assisted thoracoscopic surgery. Ann Transl Med 2015;3:111.
13. Chiniara G, Cole G, Brisbin K, et al. Simulation in healthcare: a taxonomy and a conceptual framework for instructional design and media selection. Med Teach 2013;35:e1380–95.
14. Reason J. Human error: models and management. BMJ 2000;320:768–70.
15. Ounounou E, Aydin A, Brunckhorst O, et al. Nontechnical skills in surgery: a systematic review of current training modalities. J Surg Educ 2019;76:14–24.
16. Gaba D, Fish K, Howard S, et al. Crisis management in anaesthesiology. Philadelphia: Elsevier/Saunders; 2015.
17. Boet S, Etherington N, Larrigan S, et al. Measuring the teamwork performance of teams in crisis situations: a systematic review of assessment tools and their measurement properties. BMJ Qual Saf 2019;28:327–37.
18. Arriaga AF, Bader AM, Wong JM, et al. Simulation-based trial of surgical-crisis checklists. N Engl J Med 2013;368:246–53.
19. Marshall S. The use of cognitive aids during emergencies in anesthesia: a review of the literature. Anesth Analg 2013;117:1162–71.
20. Navarro-Martínez J, Ferrero-Coloma C, Carrió-Font M, et al. Mobile applications in a crisis. Anesth Analg 2019. https://doi.org/10.1213/ANE.0000000000004137.
21. Lumb AB, Slinger P. Hypoxic pulmonary vasoconstriction: physiology and anesthetic implications. Anesthesiology 2015;122:932–46.
22. David P, Pompeo E, Fabbi E, et al. Surgical pneumothorax under spontaneous ventilation—effect on

oxygenation and ventilation. Ann Transl Med 2015;3: 106.

23. Wang M-L, Hung M-H, Chen J-S, et al. Nasal high-flow oxygen therapy improves arterial oxygenation during one-lung ventilation in non-intubated thoracoscopic surgery. Eur J Cardio Thorac Surg 2018;53:1001–6.

24. Gálvez C, Navarro-Martínez J, Bolufer S, et al. Nasal high-flow oxygen therapy during non-intubated thoracic surgery: does it offer a real advantage? Video Assist Thorac Surg 2019;4:1–5.

25. Chen K-C, Cheng Y-J, Hung M-H, et al. Nonintubated thoracoscopic surgery using regional anesthesia and vagal block and targeted sedation. J Thorac Dis 2014;6:31–6.

26. Navarro-Martínez J, Cuesta-Montero P, Ferrero-Coloma C, et al. Teaching model based on competencies: brief review and practical application in anesthesia for thoracic surgery. Rev Esp Anestesiol Reanim 2018;65:335–42.

27. Krage R, Erwteman M. State-of-the-art usage of simulation in anesthesia: skills and teamwork. Curr Opin Anaesthesiol 2015;28:727–34.

28. Navedo A, Pawlowski J, Cooper JB. Multidisciplinary and interprofessional simulation in anesthesia. Int Anesthesiol Clin 2015;53:115–33.

29. Mellin-Olsen J, Staender S, Whitaker DK, et al. The Helsinki Declaration on patient safety in anaesthesiology. Eur J Anaesthesiol 2010;27:592–7.

Team Training for Nonintubated Thoracic Surgery

Federico Tacconi, MD[a,b], Tommaso Claudio Mineo, MD[a,†],
Vincenzo Ambrogi, MD, PhD[a,b,c],*

KEYWORDS

• Learning process • Surgical training • VATS • Nonintubated thoracic surgery

KEY POINTS

- Nonintubated thoracic surgery needs a specific formation of a well-trained and close-knit staff, including surgeons, anesthesiologists, scrub nurses, operating room, and floor assistants.
- Operation requires advanced surgical skill compared with normal video-assisted thoracic surgery due to the presence of breathing or cough, patient anxiety, intolerance, or hypercapnia.
- Dry laboratory and wet laboratory training may be of scant value due to the impossibility of reproducing lung movements, whereas visiting a high-volume center or hosting an experienced team would be of greater value.
- Communication with patients, preoperatively and intraoperatively, and among the surgical team is pivotal and should follow a precise plan, reassuring the subjects, inciting them when necessary, with avoiding of impatience and anxiety.

INTRODUCTION

Nonintubated thoracic surgery consists of an operative modality where patients receive operations without orotracheal intubation and mechanical ventilation. The term, awake thoracic surgery was used in the past to indicated the same procedures, but this is not a synonym for nonintubated thoracic surgery. Indeed a vast majority of nonintubated thoracic procedures are usually performed with some degree of sedation, while preserving spontaneous breathing.[1] The spectrum of benefits of nonintubated thoracic surgery is multifaceted. It causes a global reduction in both inflammatory and metabolic stress compared with standard operations.[2] This would translate into fewer postoperative complications and, more in general, faster recovery. In addition, the authors have speculated on the intriguing possibility of the immune-depressive effect provoked by mechanical ventilation and profound anesthesia that might have a short-term impact on postoperative morbidity as well as a long-term influence on oncologic outcomes.[3]

The authors instituted the awake thoracic surgery program at the Tor Vergata University of Rome in 2000 and operations were first performed 1 year later.[4] To the best of their knowledge, this program was the first in the world to address this specific target. This program was aimed at creating a dedicated multidisciplinary unit, understanding physiologic effects of the procedures, refining surgical and anesthesiologic techniques,

Disclosure: The authors have nothing to disclose.
[a] Department of Surgical Sciences, Tor Vergata University, Via Montpellier 1, Rome 00133, Italy; [b] Division of Thoracic Surgery, Tor Vergata University Hospital, Viale Oxford 81, Rome 00133, Italy; [c] Postgraduate Training Course in Thoracic Surgery, Tor Vergata University, Rome 00133, Italy
[†] Deceased.
* Corresponding author. Department of Surgical Sciences, Tor Vergata University, Via Montpellier 1, Rome 00133, Italy.
E-mail address: ambrogi@med.uniroma2.it

Thorac Surg Clin 30 (2020) 111–120
https://doi.org/10.1016/j.thorsurg.2019.08.010

selecting patients most suitable for these procedures, and training a crescent number of specialists and nurses.

The authors' group included surgeons, anesthesiologists, intensive care physicians, physiotherapists, and both scrub and ward nurses. The authors also created a network involving external physicians, general practitioners, mass media providers, university center operators, and national health system organizations in order to popularize the progress of the program and receive adequate and reliable feedback.

All data were progressively stored in a computerized medical database in order to have readily available all demographic data, laboratory workups, imaging, informed consents, details of surgery, pathology, and follow-up data. At present, more than 1,000 cases of nonintubated video-assisted thoracic surgery (VATS) have been successfully carried out.[5]

The Department of Thoracic Surgery at Tor Vergata University is intimately attached to the Tor Vergata University School of Medicine and, at the same time, it represents the main institution of the Postgraduate School in Thoracic Surgery. Therefore, the problem of teaching the new techniques of nonintubated thoracic surgery was immediately acknowledged as critical for the institution.

THE LEARNING PROCESS

Before dealing with the practical method of teaching nonintubated surgery, the current accepted ideas about the learning process are discussed. In summary, the learning process in the humans can be classified into 2 main phases: explicit learning, where the student has the consciousness of being trained, and implicit learning, where the student has not.[6] Sequences of explicit learning are variously classified but they usually include problem-actions and effect-memories. On the contrary, implicit learning can derive from motor, temporal, and associative sequences.[7] The knowledge can be represented as decomposition into simple information and reorganization of single fragments into a hierarchical sequence.[8]

At present, the investigators of the learning process have individuated 4 different stages of competence that depict a pupil's pathway from unawareness to proficiency: unconscious incompetence, conscious incompetence, conscious competence, and finally unconscious competence (**Fig. 1**).[9] It is a well-known Socratic quotation that the first step to acquire new skill is to become aware that there are things one does not know. Inevitably, this discovery can generate a state of anxiety and unsatisfaction. Furthermore, gaining competence is not only a matter of acquiring information but also applying what has learned through testing attempts. Depending on a pupil's character, this step can also produce refusal to learn, fear to challenge, and even anger twoard the topics or against the teachers.

Acceptance and openness of the personal status are the keys to any further improvement.

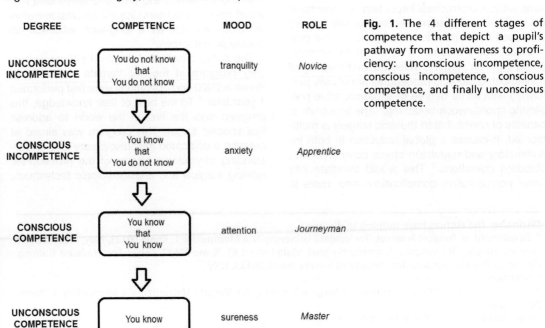

DEGREE	COMPETENCE	MOOD	ROLE
UNCONSCIOUS INCOMPETENCE	You do not know that You do not know	tranquility	*Novice*
CONSCIOUS INCOMPETENCE	You know that You do not know	anxiety	*Apprentice*
CONSCIOUS COMPETENCE	You know that You know	attention	*Journeyman*
UNCONSCIOUS COMPETENCE	You know	sureness	*Master*

Fig. 1. The 4 different stages of competence that depict a pupil's pathway from unawareness to proficiency: unconscious incompetence, conscious incompetence, conscious competence, and finally unconscious competence.

After enough practice and repetitions, with adequate effort and study, the pupil acquires proficiency. At the final stage, the ability is automatic and the actions come instinctively without aware forethought. To maintain this condition, however, continuous relearning is required, avoiding self-complacency; otherwise, the scholar might regress. Some investigators define this new status as "reflective competence level," that is, a mature recognition of personal limits paralleled by the continuous incentive toward updating.[10] Conversely, one can fall into the Dunning-Kruger effect,[11] where the incompetent cannot recognize their own incompetence. An opposite effect, the lack of self-confidence, can cause nervousness and uncertainty, affecting the performance even in a skilled individual.

There are many learning styles: verbal, visual, aural, physical, logical, social, and solitary.[12] Among these, 3 are particularly important in surgery. Verbal learning style is the most common teaching/learning style. The message is based on speech, but it is more incisive when integrated with acronyms and mnemonics and reinforced with small group conversations. Visual learning style is currently often used in surgery, especially with the introduction of videothoracoscopy popularized through materials available online. Physical learning style is effective when it comes to teach a practical topic, such as surgery. In this field, there are different patterns, discussed later. There are also, however, theoretic topics can get benefit associating movements to concepts.

THE TRAINING PROCESS

Surgical training is intimately connected to the training process. Every time a new practical process is successfully developed, the difficulty of transferring it to both authoritative senior colleagues being the same age as the teacher and to junior doctors under training should be taken into account as well. Practice needs to address weakness, and these 2 counterparts depict 2 different kind of weakness. In mature staff, there is an initial and firm hostility toward new techniques paralleled with a greater difficulty in apprenticing new movements. This burden is much more significant and scientifically proved after the age of 50 years.[13] Conversely, it is self-evident that young fellows are more keen to learn new techniques whereas they have to face their own inexperience, which becomes evident from the less brilliant surgical outcomes. This simple and intuitive statement has been recently reaffirmed by a trustworthy scientific publication.[14]

The training process in surgery has been the object of many investigations and also presents many legal and ethical issues. During a learning process, different phases are crossed that can be summarized as panic zone, learning zone, and control zone. These 3 phases must be invariably passed through, taking into mind that without feeling uncomfortable, there probably is not learning. The extent of these 3 areas changes from individual to individual, according to talent and background.

History

Due to the historical common origin from barbers, the most common form of training, if any, for surgeons was the apprenticeship.[15] Students learned surgery through direct observation and imitation of a master's actions in the operating theater or, most of the time, at a patient's home. During the nineteenth century, under the stimulus of European school, the surgeon's formation became progressively more formal and structured. On this basis, more than 1 century ago, William Stewart Halsted established the 3 main principles (**Box 1**) for training surgeons. This method produced a pyramidal-shaped selection, where from the large number of pupils starting, just a few terminated.[16] After World War II, especially in the United States, this system has been progressively reconsidered, with a definite number of pupils appointed each year, structured rotating program, precise number of years for training, and completion of the course for all applicants, outlined as a rectangular-shaped program.[17]

At the end of the millennium, the accreditation model shifted all over the world to a new one based more on interpersonal and communication

---

Box 1
Halsted's principles of surgical training

The resident must

Have intense and repetitive opportunities to take care of surgical patients under the supervision of a skilled surgical teacher

Acquire an understanding of the scientific basis of the surgical disease

Acquire skills in patient management and technical operations of increasing complexity with graded enhanced responsibility and independence

From Polavarapu HV, Kulaylat AN, Sun S, et al. 100 years of surgical education: the past, present, and future. Bull Am Coll Surg. 2013;98(7):22–7; with permission.

skills and on outcomes evaluation (**Box 2**).[18] Contemporaneously, there was increased sensitivity about the amount of resident work hours, aiming at restricting and optimizing them.[19]

Present

The introduction of minimally invasive and video-assisted surgery paralleled the Web evolution in the past few decades has considerably changed the teaching system, allowing a wider sharing of experiences and introduction of more accurate virtual reality simulators. Therefore, the chances of gaining skill in a reasonably short time before reaching the operating room have been considerably increased.[20] This rapid evolution lead to the standardization of a precise surgical pathway in the learning curve that entails progressive and more demanding movements (**Box 3**).[21] On the other hand, the faster acquisition of a skill for a new surgical technique could create the paradox of a young surgeon proficient in VATS but uncomfortable with the open access. Despite some recent studies tending to attest to the contrary,[22] there is awareness that attempting VATS without adequate training in traditional open thoracic surgery is reckless. Due to the relative diminution of open access operations, however, it is becoming more difficult to gain sufficient proficiency in all demanding steps of a trans-thoracotomy procedure.

Basically, there are 2 main systems for simulation training that are informally defined as dry laboratories and wet laboratories, which mainly signify the use of artificial-model or animal-model materials, respectively.

The dry laboratory was developed from the need for testing new technologies in a nonclinical setting. These models required the creation of virtual reality simulators.[23] Virtual reality was incorporated in some surgical training programs,[24] but unfortunately these devices in thoracic surgery have not yet reached a standard similar to those achieved in laparoscopy.[25]

Wet laboratory trainings depict somewhat more traditional programs, which use animals for the purpose of acquiring of surgical skill. They are classically divided into in vivo models, operating on living anesthetized animals, and ex vivo models, using animal tissues only. The use of animal tissues is welcomed among residents and specialists, where they can learn in a risk-free setting both basic and advanced surgical techniques, respectively. Unfortunately, due to the use of animals, wet laboratories currently are the object of ethical issues. To avoid this problem, 3-dimensntional printed Biotexture Wet Models

(BiotextureTM, FASOTEC Co., Ltd. Chiba, Japan) for surgical training have been recently developed.[26]

The interest of the major surgical companies in diffusing the newest techniques led to the implement of other forms of training. These can be categorized into preceptorship in high-volume centers and invited proctorships.[27] High-volume centers can train large numbers of apprentices in a short period of time due to the massive number of cases available every day, allowing a frequent turnover of trainees. This scheme is used for mainly trained and already employed surgeons who want to gain experience in a specific operation and avoid long absence from the work. On the contrary, invited proctorships occur when a super-expert of a defined procedure is invited to perform in a hosting institution. This allows the training of an entire team and the evaluation of the structure, protocols, materials and operations by the proctor.

NONINTUBATED SURGERY TRAINING

The title of this article clearly indicates that the training of nonintubated surgery should involve a multidisciplinary team. The development of nonintubated thoracic surgery needs a specific formation of a well-trained and close-knit staff, including surgeons, anesthesiologists, scrub nurses, operating room, and ward operators as well as psychologists and physiotherapists.

Nonintubated thoracic surgery in itself may be regarded as an evolution of standard VATS. No study so far, however, has been published regarding the learning process in this field except that from Katlic.[28] For this reason, there is no a clear-cut view of how many standard videothoracoscopic procedures should be performed before starting a nonintubated thoracic surgery program and how many nonintubated thoracic surgery procedures are necessary to reach the plateau of learning curve. Caviezel and colleagues[29] showed that, in the setting of nonintubated thoracic sympathectomy, the surgical time significantly decreases after just 4 operations performed.

Experienced Video-Assisted Thoracic Surgery Surgeons

It is assumed nowadays that a vast majority of thoracic surgery units are familiar with VATS, so that it should not be a concern to start training some easy nonintubated thoracic operations, fulfilling all the safety criteria. Nonintubated thoracic surgery, however, has its own specificities that need to be addressed. Although similar to standard VATS as far as basic technique is concerned,

Box 2
Core Accreditation Council for Graduate Medical Education competencies

1. Patient care

    Residents must be able to provide patient care that is compassionate, appropriate, and effective for the treatment of health problems and the promotion of health. Residents are expected to

    a. Communicate effectively and demonstrate caring and respectful behaviors when interacting with patients and their families

    b. Gather essential and accurate information about their patients

    c. Make informed decisions about diagnostic and therapeutic interventions based on patient information and preferences, up-to-date scientific evidence, and clinical judgment

    d. Develop and carry out patient management plans

    e. Counsel and educate patients and their families

    f. Use information technology to support patient care decisions and patient education

    g. Perform competently all medical and invasive procedures considered essential for the area of practice

    h. Provide health care services aimed at preventing health problems or maintaining health

    i. Work with health care professionals, including those from other disciplines, to provide patient-focused care

2. Medical knowledge

    Residents must demonstrate knowledge about established and evolving biomedical, clinical, and cognate (e.g., epidemiological and social-behavioral) sciences and the application of this knowledge to patient care. Residents are expected to

    a. Demonstrate an investigatory and analytic thinking approach to clinical situations

    b. Know and apply the basic and clinically supportive sciences that are appropriate to their discipline

3. Practice-based learning and improvement

    Residents must be able to investigate and evaluate their patient care practices; appraise and assimilate scientific evidence; and improve their patient care practices. Residents are expected to

    a. Analyze practice experience and perform practice-based improvement activities using a systematic methodology

    b. Locate, appraise, and assimilate evidence from scientific studies related to their patients' health problems

    c. Obtain and use information about their own population of patients and the larger population from which their patients are drawn

    d. Apply knowledge of study designs and statistical methods to the appraisal of clinical studies and other information on diagnostic and therapeutic effectiveness

    e. Use information technology to manage information, access on-line medical information, and support their own education

    f. Facilitate the learning of students and other health care professionals

4. Interpersonal and communication skills

    Residents must be able to demonstrate interpersonal and communication skills that result in effective information exchange and teaming with patients, their patients' families, and professional associates. Residents are expected to

    a. Create and sustain a therapeutic and ethically sound relationship with patients

    b. Use effective listening skills and elicit and provide information using effective nonverbal, explanatory, questioning, and writing skills

    c. Work effectively with others as members or leaders of a health care team or other professional group

5. Professionalism

Residents must demonstrate a commitment to carrying out professional responsibilities, adherence to ethical principles, and sensitivity to a diverse patient population. Residents are expected to

a. Demonstrate respect, compassion, and integrity; a responsiveness to the needs of patients and society that supersedes self-interest; accountability to patients, society, and the profession; and a commitment to excellence and continuing professional development

b. Demonstrate a commitment to ethical principles pertaining to provision or withholding of clinical care, confidentiality of patient information, informed consent, and business practices

c. Demonstrate sensitivity and responsiveness to patients' culture, age, gender, and disabilities

6. Systems-based practice

Residents must demonstrate an awareness of and responsiveness to the larger context and system of health care and the ability to effectively call on system resources to provide care that is of optimal value. Residents are expected to

a. Understand how their patient care and other professional practices affect other health care professionals, the health care organization, and the larger society and how these elements of the system affect their own practice

b. Know how types of medical practice and delivery systems differ from one another, including methods of controlling health care costs and allocating resources

c. Practice cost-effective health care and resource allocation that does not compromise quality of care

d. Advocate for quality patient care and assist patients in dealing with system complexities

e. Know how to partner with health care managers and health care providers to assess, coordinate, and improve health care and know how these activities can affect system performance

From Rose SH, Long TR, Elliott BA, et al. A historical perspective on resident evaluation, the Accreditation Council for Graduate Medical Education Outcome Project and Accreditation Council for Graduate Medical Education duty hour requirement. Anesth Analg. 2009;109(1)191; with permission.

---

the performing conditions are completely different, which may result in increased mental workload with potential for being subject to excessive physical or emotional stress to the surgeon. This is because of the following reasons: (1) the presence of breathing movements during the procedures; (2) patients may cough during the procedure; (3) patients may get anxious, intolerant, or tired during the procedures, especially if the level of sedation is insufficient; and (4) patients may develop blood gas changes that, although not necessarily hazardous, may create anxiety in the anesthesiology team, translating into further pressure on the surgeon. It is understandable that, under those circumstance, a high level of experience is needed.

Given the irreproducibility of lung and diaphragm movements, training with a simulator in a dry laboratory may be helpful only in the initial teaching phase, but it is quite useless for real learning. It is much more useful to visit a center with a high volume of nonintubated surgeries or, even better, hosting a team, at least 1 surgeon and 1 anesthesiologist expert in nonintubated operations.

As discussed previously, a high level of VATS experience is needed. Therefore, the authors recommend the following steps in order to make things smoother and limit unnecessary stress (**Box 4**). Any unnecessary waste of time should be absolutely avoided. The criteria for conversion to orotracheal intubation should be previously discussed with the anesthetist and the scrub nurse, in

---

Box 3
Core video-assisted thoracic surgery skill

Grasping and retraction—coordinated use of both hands

Cutting with instruments—alignment of cut line and instrument

Resection using endoscopic stapler—full control of the endostapler

Structure isolation and division

Anastomosis

Data from Štupnik T, Stork T. Training of video-assisted thoracoscopic surgery lobectomy: the role of simulators. Shanghai Chest 2018;2:52.

terms of both timing and intraoperative conditions. In general, it is not recommended to insist on completing the nonintubated operation if circumstances are not favorable. To establish well defined criteria for conversion to general anesthesia will give everybody in the operating room a feeling of safety.

At the beginning of nonintubated thoracic surgery learning process, it is also recommended to think liberally in terms of surgical access(es) needed to carry out the operation. Single-port technique is feasible in nonintubated anesthesia if the surgeon is already skilled with it, but it is better to initiate with operations using 2 or even 3 (but minding the excess of local anesthesia!) videothoracoscopy ports, in order to avoid any instrumental conflict that may slow the operation down.

Young Surgeons Under Training

It is desirable that nonintubated surgery can become part of any young surgeon's training, and this was included as structured agenda in the authors' postgraduate program. Due to the objective supplementary difficulties in performing this kind of surgery, however, no operation under nonintubated anesthesia should be approached without prior adequate skill in VATS acquired on intubated basis. As far as training devices is concerned, laboratory simulation may be of value in gaining ability in VATS, but proper surgical training is mandatory in centers familiar with this kind of surgery. Adequate training in nonintubated thoracic surgery should be tested with a certain number of procedures of increasing difficulty and certified at the end of the period with a specific proficiency diploma.

The authors recommend a step-by-step approach to nonintubated thoracic surgery simplified into 3 different levels of skill according to operation difficulty (**Table 1**). The ideal kinds of patients to start with are those scheduled for drainage/treatment of pleural effusion. These patients do not need relevant lung retraction, a maneuver associated with disturbing cough reflex. These patients are accustomed to lung collapse, thus highly unlikely to experience any subjective deterioration during the operation. After sufficient familiarity is gained, mediastinal mass biopsy or lung biopsy can be moved to. More difficult operations, such as resection of lung nodules or lung volume reduction surgery, can be started later in the program.

An important point to be learned is the execution of the surgical port in total absence of pain after having waited for the action of the local anesthetic and ascertained its complete effect. Conversely, there is a defined level of lidocaine that should not be overtaken and this should be accurately surveyed when accessing with more 1 port. The allowed threshold of 1% (ie, 10 mg/mL) lidocaine is less than 4.5 mg/kg: for an adult man of 75 kg, this means 337 mg, or 33.7 mL. Therefore, it is not advisable to totally inject more than three 10-mL syringes of lidocaine. The training in nonintubated surgery makes the residents considerably more skilled in performing all kinds of VATS as well as improving their capability in painless chest tube insertion at the bedside.[26]

Table 1
Road map of nonintubated video-assisted thoracic surgery for young surgeons under training

Prerequisite	Adequate Skill in Video-Assisted Thoracic Surgery Movements
Level 1	Pleural effusions drainage Pleural biopsies biportal and then uniportal Pericardial window
Level 2	Mediastinal large mass biopsy Lung biopsy Spontaneous pneumothorax Bulla resection Thoracic sympathectomy
Level 3	Mediastinal lymph node excision Wedge lung resection of nodule biportal and then uniportal Lung volume reduction

Anesthesiologist

A major part of a nonintubated procedure is based on anesthesiologist skill and specific experience. Thus, it is of paramount importance that there is an anesthesiology subunit dedicated to nonintubated thoracic surgery. Ideally, anesthesiologists who are willing to participate to a nonintubated thoracic surgery program attend any dedicated specific session. They also take part in educational and scientific activities dealing with this practice. The anesthesiology team should be aware of any specific preoperative and physiopathologic phases of nonintubated thoracic surgery, including management of surgical pneumothorax, intraoperative hypercarbia, intraoperative pain management, anxiety/panic control, and sedation. They must have documented experience in locoregional anesthesia techniques, such as thoracic epidural analgesia, paravertebral block, and others. The anesthesiology team should always be involved in the decision-making process for nonintubated thoracic surgery, either intentional or mandatory, given the high risk for general anesthesia.

Scrub Nurse

The scrub nurses are an active part of the nonintubated surgery team. They must be adequately trained and dedicated to this kind of surgery. It is important that any instrument should be ready for use in the operating room. Nonetheless, it is not necessary that any disposable tool is open, which would result in unnecessary waste of resources, but everything should be near and handy. A chest tube together with a drain chamber should be ready for use on the scrub table in order to allow rapid closure of the chest in the event of conversion to orotracheal intubation and mechanical ventilation in supine position.

In many countries, scrub nurses have permanent contracts but, unfortunately, this is not always the case. In health systems where fixed-term contracts are issued, there is high likelihood that the people in the operating room change at regular time intervals. Thus, many of the new nurses are expected to not have any experience with nonintubated thoracic surgery. This is not an ideal condition and scrub nurse should be somewhat specifically trained and tutored. Whenever this solution is impossible, it is worth spending significant time explaining exactly what nonintubated thoracic surgery consisst of and its key points in terms of operating room management.

Ward Staff

Ward staff, including physiotherapists and pain-relief therapists, should be aware of specific goals of nonintubated thoracic surgery and instructed toward this purpose with specific training. Many thoracic surgery units worldwide adopt an early recovery after surgery (ERAS) protocol, so that there is no substantial difference on how patients are managed postoperatively, regardless of the anesthesia.[30] ERAS has been shown to have substantial impact on reducing postoperative hospital stay as well as major morbidity.[31] Not adhering to ERAS principles (eg, early mobilization, fast chest tube removal, and early reprise of oral nutrition) is likely to waste and negate many of the advantages of nonintubated thoracic surgery.

Communication

Communication is a special issue in nonintubated thoracic surgery. The indication for nonintubated thoracic surgery should be carefully and fairly discussed with both patients and relatives. It also is desirable to have a psychologist involved in the team to ascertain the feasibility of the patient to bear a nonintubated or awake procedure. The scenario changes whether nonintubated thoracic surgery is offered as an intentional plan or as a mandatory strategy in patients with high risk for general anesthesia. The expected advantages and risks of nonintubated thoracic surgery should be thoroughly illustrated, ideally by providing patients with a leaflet.

Any surgical novelty brings with it its own charge of enthusiasm, which is an advantage. Conversely this enthusiasm might cause false expectations of nonintubated thoracic surgery in terms of feasibility and results. Also, there is potential for developing an unnecessary feeling of superheroism and acceptance of a challenge that may sometimes involve young and highly motivated surgeons. This kind of behavior should be absolutely counteracted by all involved staff. If patients' safety is thought to be put at risk by unwise and inappropriate application of nonintubated thoracic surgery at the side of a colleague, this should be discussed at least informally and even officially reported to lead consultant or line manager in cases of serious reiteration.

When approaching patients, language should be simple and honest enough to avoid any too much warring sentences regarding the potential risks of general anesthesia that might interfere with their decision. For those patients who accept nonintubated thoracic operations, it should be clear that despite having reasonably lesser impact on cardiac and respiratory functions, post-operative adverse events are still possible. In these patients, consent forms should clearly report the estimated likelihood of conversion to open surgery. In patients at high risk for general anesthesia, it is recommended to report the reason why the surgical treatment is preferable compared with nonsurgical options or even no treatment.

Another vital aspect is communication during surgery. Even though operating on sedated patients, during long phases of the procedure they are able to hear words and follow instructions. Therefore, it should always be borne in mind that awake patients are being operated on. Thus, a precise plan must be followed, reassuring the subjects, inciting them when necessary, avoiding expressions of impatience and anxiety, and not allowing verbal crowding. In this specific setting, intraoperative communication among the team is crucial and sensible. In particular, all comments concerning specific pathology affecting the patients as well as difficulties arising during the procedure should be avoided or at least mitigated. All these steps require an intuitive yet effective, nearly telepathic, language that necessarily implies a long common training experienced by the same team in all its components.

Implementation

Theoretically, nonintubated thoracic surgery might apply to any operation, and there are impressive reports from the literature where even massive surgeries, like esophagectomies, were done this way.[1] Nonintubated thoracic surgeries, however, are now prevalently used in the field of basic videothoracoscopic procedures, in particular, for those patients who are at increased risk of anesthesia-related complications due to cardiorespiratory comorbidity.

Despite the lack of large trials, pooled data analysis of available literature seems to show a certain advantage of nonintubated thoracic surgery in terms of postoperative hospital stay and morbidity.[32] For this reason, an increasing number of thoracic surgery centers worldwide are now interested in implementing nonintubated thoracic surgery in their practice. A survey from European Society of Thoracic Surgeons[33] showed that 69% of responders envisage an increasing adoption of nonintubated thoracic surgery in the future. Furthermore, 20% of them consider nonintubated thoracic surgery potentially feasible for any patient, regardless of the preoperative comorbidity profile.

There is some suggestion from the literature that adopting nonintubated thoracic surgery might have a positive impact on financial resources. The main factors translating into cost savings are likely the reduced incidence of postoperative adverse events. The overall procedure duration is also usually shorter—mostly because of avoidance of double-lumen intubation—a fact might that help increase the average number of operations per operating room session in the field of minor operations.[4]

Implementing nonintubated thoracic surgery might also result, however, in some sources of expenses, depending on local policies. For example, an internal audit at the authors' institution showed that there is a trend toward increased usage of locoregional anesthesia devices in the nonintubated thoracic surgery group. So the authors' policy now is to prefer ultrasound-guided, single-shot paravertebral or erector spinae block instead of catheterization whenever clinically appropriate.

Costs for training and maintaining of skill are difficult to calculate, but, reasonably, in many countries there is no substantial adjunctive burden in implementing nonintubated thoracic surgery inside an ordinary clinical practice, unless clinical fellowship contracts are needed for this specific purpose.

The authors suggest that proficiency in nonintubated thoracic surgery should be certified and listed as a credential in submitting applications for surgical positions. Certification in nonintubated surgery also should be issued to operating room staff, including dedicated thoracic anesthesiologists, scrub nurses, and technicians. Commitment to maintain the same team for at least 40 procedures a year also should be provided by the administration.[34] Another important point for implementation is the exchange of data, experience, and professional figures within the different institutions.

SUMMARY

Nonintubated surgery is one of the novel frontiers in thoracic surgery. Thoracic surgeons who are willing to introduce this kind of surgery in their unit should be aware of specific technical and managerial problems of this surgery. Training in nonintubated surgery deserves a proper pathway. The authors recommend a step-by-step approach as well as an established experience on traditional VATS.

Communication with patient, preoperatively and intraoperatively, and among the surgical team is pivotal and should follow a precise plan reassuring the subjects and encouraging them when necessary, with avoidance of impatience and anxiety. Nothing can be done without continuous educational and human exchanges.

REFERENCES

1. Mineo TC, Tacconi F. From "awake" to "monitored anesthesia care" thoracic surgery. A 15 year evolution. Thorac Cancer 2014;5:1–13.
2. Tacconi F, Pompeo E, Sellitri F, et al. Surgical stress hormones response is reduced after awake videothoracoscopy. Interact Cardiovasc Thorac Surg 2010;10:666–71.
3. Mineo TC, Sellitri F, Vanni G, et al. Immunological and inflammatory impact of non-intubated lung metastasectomy. Int J Mol Sci 2017;18:1466.
4. Pompeo E, Mineo D, Rogliani P, et al. Feasibility and results of awake thoracoscopic resection of solitary pulmonary nodules. Ann Thorac Surg 2004;78:1761–8.
5. Mineo TC, Tamburini A, Perroni G, et al. 1000 cases of tubeless video-assisted thoracic surgery at the Rome Tor Vergata University. Future Oncol 2016; 12(23S):13–8.
6. Graf P, Schacter DL. Implicit and explicit memory for new associations in normal and amnesic subjects. J Exp Psychol Learn Mem Cogn 1985;11:501–18.
7. Dominey P. Complex sensory-motor sequence learning based on recurrent state representation and reinforcement learning. Biol Cybern 1995;73:265–74.
8. Bat-Sheva E, Reif F. Effects of knowledge organization on task performance. Cogn Instr 1984;1:5–44.
9. Broadwell MM. Teaching for learning (XVI). The Gospel Guardian 1969;20(41):1–3a.
10. Taylor B. Reflective practice. Philadelphia: Buckingham, Open University Press; 2000.
11. Kruger J, Dunning D. Unskilled and unaware of it: how difficulties in recognizing one's own incompetence lead to inflated self-assessments. J Pers Soc Psychol 1999;77:1121–34.
12. Smith DM, Kolb DA. User's guide for the learning-style inventory: a manual for teachers and trainers. Boston: McBer and Co; 1996.
13. Coats RO, Wilson AD, Snapp-Childs W, et al. The '50s cliff: perceptuo-motor learning rates across the lifespan. PLoS One 2014;9(1):e85758.
14. Birkmeyer JD, Finks JF, O'Reilly A, et al. Surgical skill and complication rates after bariatric surgery. N Engl J Med 2013;369:1434–42.
15. Dobson J, Walker RM. Barbers and barber-surgeons of London: a history of the barbers' and barber-surgeons companies. Oxford (United Kongdom): Blackwell Scientific Publ; 1979.
16. Halsted WS. The training of the surgeon. Bull Johns Hopkins Hosp 1904;15:267–75.
17. Sealy WC. Halsted is dead: time for change in graduate surgical education. Curr Surg 1999;56:34–9.
18. Rose SH, Long TR, Elliott BA, et al. A historical perspective on resident evaluation, the Accreditation Council for Graduate Medical Education Outcome Project and Accreditation Council for Graduate Medical Education duty hour requirement. Anesth Analg 2009;109:190–3.
19. Davis EC, Risucci DA, Blair PG, et al. Women in surgery residency programs: evolving trends from a national perspective. J Am Coll Surg 2011;212:320–6.
20. Dunkin B, Adrales GL, Apelgren K, et al. Surgical simulation: a current review. Surg Endosc 2007;21:357–66.
21. Štupnik T, Stork T. Training of video-assisted thoracoscopic surgery lobectomy: the role of simulators. Shanghai Chest 2018;2:52.
22. Billé A, Okiror L, Harrison-Phipps K, et al. Does previous surgical training impact the learning curve in video-assisted thoracic surgery lobectomy for trainees? Thorac Cardiovasc Surg 2016;64:343–7.
23. Haluck RS, Satava RM, Fried G, et al. Establishing a simulation center for surgical skills: what to do and how to do it. Surg Endosc 2007;21:1223–32.
24. Solomon B, Bizekis C, Dellis SL, et al. Simulating video-assisted thoracoscopic lobectomy: a virtual reality cognitive task simulation. J Thorac Cardiovasc Surg 2011;141:249–55.
25. Bedetti B, Schnorr P, Schmidt J, et al. The role of wet lab in thoracic surgery. J Vis Surg 2017;3:61.
26. Morikawa T, Yamashita M, Odaka M, et al. A step-by-step development of real size chest model for simulation of thoracoscopic surgery. Interact Cardiovasc Thorac Surg 2017;25:173–6.
27. Sandri A, Sihoe ADL, Salati M, et al. Training in uniportal video-assisted thoracic surgery. Thorac Surg Clin 2017;27:417–23.
28. Katlic MR. Video-Assisted Thoracic Surgery utilizing local anesthesia and sedation: how I teach it. Ann Thorac Surg 2017;104:727–30.
29. Caviezel C, Schuepbach R, Grande B, et al. Establishing a non-intubated thoracoscopic surgery program for bilateral uniportal sympathectomy. Swiss Med Wkly 2019;149:w20064.
30. Semenkovich TR, Hudson JL, Subramianian M, et al. Enhanced Recovery After Surgery (ERAS) in thoracic surgery. Semin Thorac Cardiovasc Surg 2018;30:342–9.
31. Batchelor TJP, Ljungqvist O. A surgical perspective of ERAS guidelines in thoracic surgery. Curr Opin Anaesthesiol 2019;32:17–22.
32. Tacconi F, Pompeo E. Non-intubated video-assisted thoracic surgery: where does evidence stand? J Thorac Dis 2016;8:S364–75.
33. Pompeo E, Sorge R, Akopov A, et al. Non-intubated thoracic surgery: a survey from the European Society of Thoracic Surgeons. Ann Transl Med 2015;3:37.
34. Mineo TC, Ambrogi V. Awake thoracic surgery for secondary spontaneous pneumothorax: another advancement. J Thorac Cardiovasc Surg 2012;144:1533–4.

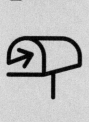

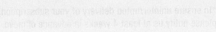

Printed and bound by CPI Group (UK) Ltd, Croydon, CR0 4YY

08/05/2025

01864745-0016